THE HARVONI EXPERIENCE:

How I beat HEPATITIS C in 12 weeks with one pill a day

- My 12-week Harvoni Journal and Research
- Candid Treatment Experiences of Many Users
- Brief History of the Hepatitis C Virus
- HCV/RNA, ALT, ADT, Viral Loads Explained
- Which drugs work for Genotypes 1,2,3,4,5,6
- Harvoni, Epclusa, Solvadi , Zepatier, Dazlinza
- Options in Paying for Treatment
- How to Lessen Severity of Side Effects
- Alternative Treatments & Lifestyle Changes
- Hepatitis C Resources, Websites, Contacts

By
Valerie and Banning Lary, PhD

THE HARVONI EXPERIENCE:

How I beat HEPATITIS C in 12 weeks with one pill a day

Published by:
Promedion
P. O. Box 365
Lexington, KY 40588 U. S. A.

Dazlinza® is a registered trademark of Bristol-Myers Squibb.
Harvoni®, Sovaldi ® and Epclusa® are registered trademarks of Gilead Sciences, Inc.
Zepatier® is a registered trademark of Merck & Company.

While every effort has been made to assure the accuracy and authenticity of the contents of this book, the authors make no guarantees that what is stated in this book will work for you. The authors are not medical doctors and are not licensed to provide medical advice. We advise every person to research the information contained in this book for themselves and verify it with their physician of choice. The essence of quoted responses from Hep C patients is real, though the content has been altered for reasons of privacy and anonymity. We invite your comments.
comments@theharvoniexperience.com

Publisher's Cataloging-in-Publication Data
Names: Lary, Valerie. | Lary, Banning K.
Title: The Harvoni experience: how I beat hepatitis C in 12 weeks with one pill a day / Valerie Lary [and] Banning K. Lary, PhD.
Description: Lexington, KY : Promedion, 2016. | Includes bibliographical references.
Identifiers: ISBN 978-1-885832-47-4 (pbk.) | ISBN 978-1-885832-46-7 (ebook)
Subjects: LCSH: Hepatitis C--Treatment. | Hepatitis C--Patients--Anecdotes. | Hepatitis C--Popular works. | Antiviral agents--Therapeutic use. | Chronic diseases--Psychological aspects. | MESH: Hepatitis C--drug therapy. | Hepatitis C--psychology--United States--autobiography. | BISAC: HEALTH & FITNESS / Diseases / Contagious.
Classification: LCC RC848.H425 L37 2016 (print) | LCC RC848.H425 (ebook) | DDC 616.3/623--dc23.

Printed in the United States of America
By Promedion Professional Medical Education, Lexington, KY 40588

10 9 8 7 6 5 4 3 2 1

This book is dedicated to my soul mate, my daughters and my grand daughters who have given me the inspiration to live.

*   *   *

And, a special thanks to all those who shared their experiences with me, in person, through emails and in the online chat rooms and support groups. I hope your treatments are successful and your cures permanent.

THE HARVONI EXPERIENCE:

How I beat HEPATITIS C in 12 weeks with one pill a day

CONTENTS

PREFACE – Undetected!

In the weeks leading up to my Harvoni treatment, I had many questions. Would I have any energy? Would I be able to work? Would I get angry or depressed? Would my hair fall out? Would it affect the way I dealt with my loved ones and friends? Would I experience fatigue, cramps, headaches or other possible side effects cited in the product literature? Would it affect my sex drive?

I'll never forget the words my doctor said when she read the results of my blood panel on the 84th day during the post treatment office visit: "Your levels are less than 15. In other words undetected!" I felt like I was floating above the carpet. The Harvoni had worked! The Hepatitis C virus was not discernable in my blood sample. In essence, I had beaten the disease and I could have a normal life. No longer would I live in fear that my time on earth might end at any day, that my soul mate would have to go on without me, that I would never see my children fully blossom into adulthood, or see my grandchildren grow up, finish school and find mates.

WEEK (scheduled)	Screen	Baseline	1	2	3	4	6	8	12
DATE (scheduled)		5/10/16	5/17/16	5/24/16	5/31/16	6/7/16	6/21/16	7/5/16	8/2/16
WEEK (actual)		0.0	1.0	2.0	3.0	3.9	6.0	8.0	12.0
DATE (actual)	4/19/16	5/10/16	5/17/16	5/24/16	5/31/16	6/6/16	6/21/16	7/5/16	8/2/16
Harvoni		400/90	400/90	400/90	400/90	400/90	400/90	400/90	400/90
HCV RNA	4,600,000	4,660,000		<15		n.d.			n.d.

This book is the story of my twelve weeks of Harvoni treatment, and first month post treatment, mixed in with the unvarnished experiences of my fellow "dragon slayers" along the path toward freedom from the virus. This book also contains as much current factual information we could find about Hepatitis C, alternative treatment options, and data from scientific publications. I say "we" as my story would not be possible without the help of my soul mate of thirty years, a brilliant researcher and writer with a PhD in psychology, who suggested I keep a journal to use as the backbone for this story, who coached me, and was there for me every step of the way. Thank you, Dr. B!

We have purposefully made this book short and to the point, so others can read the information in a couple hours instead of having to sift through a lot of extraneous data and verbiage they wouldn't use or remember. Our goal was to present everything we wanted to know before I started treatment in a concise and easy to read format. We hope you will find this book informative and that it will help alleviate some of the fears and worries you might have about taking Harvoni.

Knowledge silences ignorance. Godspeed!

I Have Hepatitis C

I didn't know I had Hepatitis C until about seven years ago, though the virus had been living in my body for almost forty years. I was feeling unusually tired and, even though I was getting older, I didn't seem to have the energy or mental clarity I should have. So, I went to see the doctor and knew something was wrong by the look on his face.

"Did you know your liver enzymes are extremely elevated?" he asked.

"No." I didn't know what liver enzymes were. I studied and found that enzymes are biocatalysts which facilitate every chemical reaction in your body, such as the breakdown of food in the digestive system, so it can be more readily absorbed by the cells. When a liver is damaged it leaks more enzymes than are necessary for body balance, or homeostasis. Further:

"Liver enzymes are indicated in a blood test by a liver panel, a group of tests gastroenterologists use to detect and evaluate liver damage or disease. The liver's primary functions are to metabolize and detoxify harmful substances in the body. The liver can be inflamed through an infection such as hepatitis, or scarred by cirrhosis. A liver panel measures levels of enzymes, proteins and other substances "produced, processed or eliminated by the liver." [1]

The individual tests in the blood panel measure such substances as Alanine aminotransferase (ALT), Akaline phosphatase (ALP), Aspartate aminotransferase (AST), Bilirubin, Albumin, Total protein (TP), and others.

"Your AST is 147, normal is 10 to 40," said my doctor. "Your ALT is 162, normal is 7 to 56."

	Screen
WEEK (scheduled)	
DATE (scheduled)	
WEEK (actual)	
DATE (actual)	4/16/16
Harvoni	
HCV RNA	4,500,000
WBC	5.5
Hemoglobin	13.7
Platelets	149
AST	147
ALT	162
Alkaline Phosphatase	67

"What does that mean?"

"It means your liver may be infected with the Hepatitis C virus and you may have the beginnings of cirrhosis. We need to get a liver biopsy to be sure."

I could hardly breathe. I had heard horror stories about Hep C. I had friends who died in their forties from it. My father had died of liver disease at age 62. I felt the cold squeeze of death come over me and started to shake.

"What can I do?" I asked, my eyes filling with tears.

"Stop drinking alcohol and smoking cigarettes to start."

But, I liked drinking and smoking. Getting a buzz was the only time I felt good any more.

"And, change your diet," he said. "Cut out red meat. Exercise more and drink lots of water."

"What about treatment?"

"There's Interferon. But, it's hard to get approved and it's very expensive. And, it has been proven to be effective only about 50% of the time."

I knew a hair stylist who took Interferon for Hep C. She had to administer injections and take pills for nine months. It was like chemotherapy. She was often nauseous, weak and depressed, and couldn't go to work. She lost so much weight she looked like a skeleton. And, all her hair fell out. That wasn't for me.

"Is that the only option?"

"Some people try alternative treatments like herbs and acupuncture, but I haven't heard of a case where that worked to cure Hep C."

"No other drugs are available?"

"I hear they are working on it, but it won't be for years," the doctor said, dashing my hopes that a safe rapid cure was possible.

I left the office feeling like my life as I had known it was over. I felt hopeless and could not confront the realization that my death was imminent. I fell into a deep depression, went home and drank myself to sleep. When the liver biopsy results came back, the doctor told me I had cirrhosis and that "your liver is shot." He looked at me like,

"You're done. Next!" He had the worst bedside manner of any doctor I had ever heard of. The way he wrote my diagnosis on a posted note slip made me feel like I was some kind of demented animal.

My soul mate noticed something had changed about me and asked if anything was wrong, but it took me several weeks to finally tell him. We had been sleeping together for years, had two lovely children and shared everything. I felt guilty that I may have passed the virus on to him without knowing it. Or, may even have given it to my daughters. Thankfully, we later found that this had not happened and that the virus belonged to me alone.

I told him and we hugged and cried together for an afternoon, talking about our options and how we had to change our lives. But, really nothing could be changed. We couldn't afford Interferon and I didn't want to go through the experience any way. So, for the next seven years I tried pharmaceutical drugs and drank alcohol to try and escape my fate. I was an old rock-n-roller who had lived in the fast lane, knowing intimately some of the top artists in rock history. I thought it would be better to burn out than to waste away. I wasn't going to sit by and succumb to some stupid disease. I would take myself out before the disease could do it.

I know that must sound crazy, but the Hep C virus had that effect on my thinking and behavior. I really didn't care if I lived or died and just wanted to have a good time while it lasted. My choices in those days were not the best, I admit, and I know I messed up some good relationships for which I am sorry. But, Hep C, as I was later to discover, is often responsible for a severe decline in brain function known as Hepatic Encephalopathy, caused by a build-up of toxins in the blood the liver cannot adequately remove. The distress in my body caused the aberration in my thinking.[2]

So, life went on like this for six years, knowing the Hep C virus was eating me up from the inside. I had horrible mood swings and erratic behavior. I hardly ever had a day where I felt normal, whatever that was. People regarded me as being unpredictable. The fights with my mate and children became more dramatic and frequent, exacerbated by financial problems. But, no need to go into all of that. It is too personal and painful. But, those of you reading this can probably relate.

A couple years later we moved to a smaller place, but the excitement and newness of the location wore off quickly. All the color and joy had been bleached out of my life by the disease and my subsequent behavior. I was no longer interested in intimacy with my mate. My relationships with my daughters and friends became strained. My life of quiet desperation continued for several interminable years.

And, then, a ray of light appeared. Reports of a new drug coming on the market that could cure Hep C in 90 days with few side effects would soon be available. It was called Harvoni®. But, it would take finding a new doctor and great timing for me to be able to obtain treatment.

What is Hepatitis C?

As of this writing (September 2016) a reported 130-150 million people in the world have chronic Hepatitis C infection and, ironically, most do not know it. A significant number of these will develop cirrhosis or liver cancer and about 700,000 each year will die from related diseases.[1] In the United States, the Centers for Disease Control and Prevention estimate 2.7 to 3.9 million people have chronic Hep C, with over 30,000 new cases of acute Hep C being reported annually. About 75% to 85% of acute cases will develop into chronic Hep C.[2] Acute refers to the short term illness that occurs within the first six months of exposure. Chronic Hepatitis C is a long-term illness which can become progressively worse over time and lead to cirrhosis (scarring of the liver) or liver cancer which can result in death.

Having HCV put me in a group that contains about 2% of the U. S. population, including regular people and famous ones alike. When I began to research, I ran across several sites where well-known people were mentioned who had become infected with HCV by different means and the treatments they used. One of the most notable was country singer Naomi Judd, who became infected by a needle stick when working as an intensive care unit nurse in the 1980s.

Naomi was living the dream of a rock star, traveling the world and performing to packed houses with her daughter Wynonna, when she began to experience debilitating muscle aches and fatigue, leading to panic attacks and depression. "I became incredibly ill to the point where I couldn't even brush my teeth or change my nightgown," she said.[3]

At the time she was diagnosed, the only medical treatment available was Interferon, with a 15% cure rate. Naomi injected the drug into her stomach three times a week, and adopted a holistic approach to healing, integrating acupuncture, meditation and other alternative practices including a more plant-based diet. She bravely struggled to fight off the disease for a long time before meeting Dr. Bruce Bacon, of the St. Louis University Liver Center (Missouri), who put her on a newer Interferon regimen which eventually cured her of the disease. Her book, *Naomi's Breakthrough Guide: 20 Choices to Transform Your Life,* details the steps she took to beat the Hep C virus and return her to a normal life. Today, Naomi, whose duo albums with Wynona have won five Grammys and eight Country Music Association awards, is a vocal spokeswoman for health and HCV awareness.[3]

Rock legend Steven Tyler suffered the symptoms of Hep C for years before he took a break from Aerosmith and sought Interferon treatment he equates to chemotherapy. "I would put the kids to sleep then wake up at 3 in the morning with a nosebleed," he said, discussing the toll treatment took on his body and marriage. Tyler says many people who have Hep C don't know it. "It's the silent killer," he says.[4]

Pamela Anderson, flamboyant personality, star of "Baywatch" and movies, reported being "cured" of Hep C in 2015 after living with the virus for 16 years.[5]

Unlikely crooner and star of "Gomer Pyle" Jim Nabors, lived with a compromised immune system from Hep C after becoming infected during a liver transplant.[6] An extensive article in Wikipedia lists many celebrities who have battled Hep C, including singers David Crosby and Lou Reed, and porn star Linda Lovelace.[7]

Actor, singer, dancer Danny Kaye, who was big in the 1940s, '50s and '60s, starring in such films as "The Secret Life of Walter Mitty" (1946) and "The Inspector General" (1948), became infected with Hep C from a blood transfusion during surgery and died four years later.[8]

Other high profile people who have had Hep C include stunt dare devil Evel Knievel, who became infected with a blood transfusion following one his many crashes.[9] James Earl Ray, confessed assassin of civil rights leader Martin Luther King, died in prison of complications brought on by Hep C.[10] Comedian Robert Schimmel came in to contact with HCV from a blood transfusion while serving in the Air Force.[11]

Existentialistic novelist Hubert Selby, Jr. (*Last Exit to Brooklyn, Requiem for a Dream*) caught Hep C while receiving treatment for tuberculosis.[12] Ken Kesey (*One Flew Over the Cuckoo's Nest, Sometimes a Great Notion*), hero of Tom Wolfe's *The Electric Kool-Aid Acid Test,* died of liver cancer brought on by HCV.[13] Nik Cohn popular music journalist and critic, said that having hepatitis C was like "having permanent jet lag."[14]

In sports, American professional wrestler, Billy Graham, claims to have gotten HCV from "rolling around in the ring in other wrestler's blood."[15] Pro football place kicker, Rolf Benirschke, became infected by blood transfusions during treatment for ulcerative colitis.[16] And, New York Yankees baseball legend Mickey Mantle died from metastasized cancer that spread from his liver in 1995.[17]

Pathologist, Dr. Jack Kervorkian, who served eight years in prison for actions stemming from his role as champion of terminal patient's "right to die," claimed he came into contact with the Hep C virus while testing blood for transfusions during the Vietnam War.[18]

Robert. F. Kennedy, Jr, son of the slain Attorney General, was treated with Interferon while in rehab for alcoholism in 1983.[19] Japanese businessman, Rocky Aoki, former Olympic wrestler, powerboat racing champion, and flashy founder of the Benihana restaurant chain, died in 2008 due to liver failure brought on by HCV and cirrhosis. His motto was "You afraid of dying, you afraid of living also."[20]

One of the best uses of celebrity is to use fame to help create awareness of the disease that once sapped their energy and decimated their lives. R & B artist Natalie Cole and country rock legend Greg Allman, both long term sufferers of HCV, gave a benefit concert in New York that raised over $250,000 to help spread awareness of the disease and help remove the social stigma through the "Tune in to Hep C," a national campaign sponsored by Merck and the American Liver foundation. [21]

Hepatitis C does not discriminate between rich and poor, famous or ordinary, male or female. It is a disease that can infect anyone anywhere who is unfortunate enough to come into contact with the debilitating virus that can lead to sickness, degradation of quality of life and eventual death.

Hepatitis literally means 'inflammation of the liver' and refers to a family of viral infections that affect the health and functioning of the liver. The liver is an essential organ which helps purify the blood by neutralizing the harmful and toxic effects of chemicals such as medications and alcohol. The liver also produces essential proteins, such as albumin, that keep the body healthy and promote rapid blood clotting in case of an injury. Sugars, fats and vitamins are stored in the liver for transport through the blood stream to where they are needed to rebuild the body and promote rapid healing. The liver is also responsible for changing the state of harmful chemicals, such as ammonia or bilirubin, so they can be eliminated in the urine or stool.[22] When liver function is hampered by excessive alcohol use or Hepatitis, it cannot perform as needed, resulting in signs and symptoms described throughout this book.

No one knows exactly where Hepatitis C came from, as there are no stored blood samples older than 50 years that can be tested for the virus. Virologists (people who study viruses) conjecture that Hepatitis C may have been around for thousands of years evolving into its current genotype strains. Other experts speculate HCV may have originated with primates 35 million years ago, or the different subtypes from people who lived 500 years ago in West Africa. However, since HCV is mainly spread via blood-to-blood contact, and since different strains are found in remote areas all over the world, the scientific facts suggest HCV has been on earth for a long time.[23]

While scientists had developed blood tests to identify hepatitis B (1963) and hepatitis A (1973), the hepatitis C virus was not specifically identified by investigators from the Centers for Disease Control and Chiron until 1989.

Transfusions were found to be a main method of infection, and HCV screening for donors began in 1990. By 1992 blood tests were perfected which virtually eliminated

HCV from the blood supply – a key year in the history of the disease.[23]

The most common viral strains are Hepatitis A, B and C, although D, E, and a possible G have been identified. Hep A, B, and C all start as infections contacted primarily by coming into close person-to-person contact with an infected person, from contact with infected blood, semen or other bodily fluids or via birth from an infected mother. Common known ways of disease transmission include sharing needles during drug use, piercings, tattoos, sexual contact, ingestion of infected fecal matter (as in an unclean restaurant or food stand), sexual contact, and from organ transplants or blood transfusions usually before 1992. Travel to areas of the world where high rates of the virus are known increase the possibility of infection.[1,2,23]

Hepatitis is a blood-born virus, meaning it cannot be spread through sneezing, hugging, kissing, using another's spoon, fork or glass unless blood is present. However, it can be spread by using another's razor, toothbrush, nail clippers and so forth if they have come into contact with an infected person's blood and have not been sterilized.

Initial symptoms from acute (short-term) Hepatitis A, B, and C are similar, though can vary in complexity and intensity: fatigue, dark urine, light-colored stools, fever, jaundice, nausea, loss of appetite, joint pain, diarrhea, abdominal pain, vomiting and other flu-like symptoms. The symptoms from HAV usually do not develop past the acute stage, and people with healthy immune systems recover without additional complications. Once you become infected with HAV and your body processes internal treatment, you cannot get it again. HBV is much more severe than HAV, especially among infants who contract the disease from their infected mothers, with up to 90% experiencing chronic symptoms at birth. Most people with acute HBV recover, though 15% to 20% of chronically infected persons develop cirrhosis, liver failure or liver cancer. Drugs are being developed to thwart the spread of HBV within the body, but do not eliminate the virus.[2,23] The best protection against contracting Hepatitis A and B is vaccination, however there is no known vaccine to prevent Hepatitis C infection, and must be dealt with after a person gets tested and undergoes treatment.

Hepatitis C (HCV) is by far the most potentially lethal strain of the virus and the most difficult to stop. A person can never say he or she is 'cured' of HCV. A trace of the virus will always remain even though reported viral loads are 'undetected' and HCV/RNA blood test numbers have returned to within the normal range. As HCV is a worldwide phenomenon, different varieties of the virus have been discovered relative to the geographical location where the person became infected. This is often a clue about when a person contracted the disease and by what method. In my case, I believe I became infected in Melbourne, Australia, around 1975 at a rock concert where they had ear piercing booths. I remember thinking at the time if the guy who did the piercing had used a clean needle. But, I was ignorant in those days of Hepatitis, never knowing that one innocent act could come back to haunt me years later.

While there are different types of Hepatitis (A, B, C, D, E, etc.), within HCV there are also different ranges of the virus identified by their 'genotype' and 'subtype.' Determining what genotype of the virus you have is essential in selecting the right treatment protocol, including what drugs may be most effective in attacking and eradicating the virus from your bodily system.[24,25]

An easy way to understand genotypes is by using the analogy of dogs. There are many types of dogs, each breed with a certain combination of unique characteristics. A brown and white Jack Russell terrier with its short legs and short hair is far different from the wide-bodied thick-limbed longhaired St. Bernard, for example. Within the terrier class you have the Jack Russell, but also the fluffy English Bedlington Terrier, the tiny Australian Terrier and the American Staffordshire Terrier, also known as the 'pit bull.' These breeds have evolved in different geographical locations over the centuries from the common ancestor of the grey wolf, much like the different genotypes of the Hep C virus have evolved into geographic specific genotypes and subtypes:

1a – mostly found in North & South America; also common in Australia.
1b – mostly found in Europe and Asia.
2a – is the most common genotype 2 in Japan and China.
2b – is the most common genotype 2 in the U.S. and Northern Europe.
2c – the most common genotype 2 in Western and Southern Europe.
3a – highly prevalent in Australia and South Asia.
4a – prevalent in Egypt.
4c – prevalent in Central Africa.
5a – prevalent only in South Africa.
6a – restricted to Hong Kong, Macau and Vietnam.
7a and 7b – rare, found in Thailand and the Congo.
8a, 8b & 9a – prevalent in Vietnam.
10a & 11a – found in Indonesia.[26]

In a recent comprehensive study of HCV genotypes present in 117 countries, researchers found that "genotype 1 is the most prevalent worldwide, comprising 83.4 million cases (46.2% of all HCV cases), approximately one-third of which are in East Asia. Genotype 3 is the next most prevalent globally (54.3 million, 30.1%); genotypes 2, 4, and 6 are responsible for a total 22.8% of all cases; genotypes 5, 7, 8, 9, 10 and 11 comprise the remaining <1%. While genotypes 1 and 3 dominate in most countries irrespective of economic status, the largest proportions of genotypes 4 and 5 are in lower-income countries."[27] In the United States, approximately 75% of the people infected with HCV have genotype 1, 20-25% have genotypes 2 or 3, and the remainder having genotypes 4,5 and 6.[28]

It follows then, that I would be diagnosed with genotype '1a' as I spent my early years living in Australia. It is the estimated that of the 160,000 Australians with HCV, approximately 35% have subtype '1a', 15% have '1b', 7% have '2', 35% have '3' (mostly being 3a), the others having a mixture of other genotypes as they possibly had contracted the virus from other countries. Thus, having HCV genotype '1a,' my doctor was able to pinpoint the brand of drug that would be most effective in fighting my strain of the virus: Harvoni.

HARVONI AND OTHER HCV DRUGS

Pharmaceutical companies have been active in the past few years developing and licensing drugs that attack and stop the advance of the Hepatitis C virus without the horrible side effects of interferon. The antiviral properties of interferon, a naturally occurring substance in the human body, was discovered by scientists in 1957. It was named interferon due to its abilities to 'interfer' with viral replication, and found to exist in three identifiable types – alpha, beta and gamma. Interferon alpha, (Shering's Intron A) was the first brand product approved to treat hepatitis C by the FDA in 1991, with different versions approved in 1996 (Roche/Genentech Roferon A) and 1997 (Amgen/InterMune-Infergen).[1,2] The initial treatment protocol was to inject 3 million units of interferon alpha, three times a week for 48 weeks. Sustained virologic response (SVR) rates – negative viral load 6 months post-treatment), were only 9% for genotype 1 and 30% for genotypes 2 and 3. The addition of ribavirin to the treatment regimen in 1998 was found to produce a synergy which enhanced treatment outcomes, doubling or tripling SVR post-treatment results.[2]

Interferon, with or without the anti-viral drug ribavirin, was for years virtually the only effective medical treatment option, despite the length of treatment, horrible side effects and a curtailed ability to function normally. Frequent injections were necessary as interferon was broken down by the body, usually within 12 to 24 hours, leaving little interferon to kill or suppress HVC.[2] An improved type of interferon marketed under the brand name Pegagsys®, was approved by the FDA in 2002 and is usually administered with Copegus® (ribavirin) tablets. Pegylation attaches biologically inert polyethylene glycol strands to the interferon molecule, prolonging its effectiveness by slowing the breakdown and elimination rate, thus keeping it in the bloodstream longer to fight the virus and increase the likelihood of SVR.[2]

Pegagsys® (*peginterferon alfa-2a*), manufactured by Genetech and approved by the FDA in 2002, is a type of interferon, a protein (cytokine) made by the body to fight off infections, such as flu viruses.[1] As the Hepatitis C virus is basically invisible to the immune system, the amount of interferon naturally produced is not enough to attack and kill the disease. Thus, supplementary injections of synthetic interferon are used to help healthy cells detect and defend against the virus, help the immune system stop the virus from multiplying, and help the body remove infected white cells. Treatment programs can run six to twelve months.[2] Pegasys® can be administered alone or with Copegus® (ribavirin) tablets, also FDA approved in 2002. "Patients in clinical studies, including genotypes 1-4, had a better than 50 percent change of reducing HCV to undetectable levels."[3] Females who are pregnant, or who plan to become pregnant, and their male partners are warned not to take Pegasys® with or without Copegus® as the risk of birth defects is increased.

Side effects from synthetic interferon can include problems with blood, thyroid, blood sugar, eyes, liver, nerves, or lungs; inflammation of pancreas and intestines; serious allergic reactions and skin reactions; insomnia, fatigue and irritability; headaches and body aches; decreased appetite, weight loss, nausea and vomiting; depression and mood changes; decreased white blood cells and platelets; difficulty concentrating and impaired memory; and, effect on growth in children.[3]

Like many people, I felt undergoing the rigors of interferon + ribavirin with its 50% "cure rate" for certain genotypes, was not worth the trouble due to the pronounced side effects and length of treatment. For years I have been trying to find some kind of alternative treatment such as herbs, acupuncture, dietary changes, faith healers – anything but having to take interferon. Some herbalists recommended milk thistle (*Silybum marianum* or *sillymarin*), so I tried it and it seemed to make me feel worse. Others recommended zinc, colloidal silver, probiotics, yoga, qigong, vitamin D, green tea, colonic flushes and other detox methods. None of them worked. This fact was born out by medical research.[4,5]

The cold reality was, there was NOT any other cure except the intense interferon / ribavirin regimen which was only effective half the time. That meant half the people who underwent the brutal treatment did it for nothing. Drug makers clearly understood the potential advantages and profitability of finding a speedier remedy with fewer side effects, and sought to develop or license effective products. Between 2011 and 2016, the Federal Food and Drug Administration (FDA), the oversight agency charged with protecting the health of consumers in the United States, approved a slate of new drugs which quickly found their way to market under these trade names: Incivek®, Victrelis®, Olysio®, Viekira Pak®, Sovaldi®, Harvoni®, Technivie®, Daklinza®, Zepatier®, and Epclusa®.[6] All of these drugs are administered by daily tablets instead of injections, except those used in conjunction with peginterferon alfa (Incivek and Victrelis).

A brief summary of each medication follows, information drawn from drug package inserts and FDA reports posted online. For more detailed information, click on the links in the reference section at the end of the book, or search the drug names on Google as new studies are posted every week. FDA.gov is always a good source of the latest verifiable information about new drug approvals and problems. Your medical doctor will determine which drug is right for you, considering such factors as HCV genotype, age, gender, ethnicity, pregnancy, and whether or not you are "treatment-naïve," (not having undergone previous HCV treatment), or "treatment experienced" (having undergone previous treatment that was unsuccessful).

Incivek® (*telaprevir*), manufactured by Vertex was approved by the FDA 2011 for use "in combination with pegainterferon alfa and ribavirin, for the treatment of genotype 1 chronic hepatitis C with compensated liver disease in adult patients [some level of damage to the liver but the liver still functions], including cirrhosis [scarring of the liver], who are treatment-naïve, or who have been previously treated with interferon-based treatment, including prior null responders, partial responders and relapsers."[7] Incivek must not be used as a stand-alone monotherapy, but must be used in conjunction with interferon and ribavirin. Incivek tablets are administered twice daily 10-14 hours apart with food (not low fat) for 12 weeks, followed by a response-guided regimen of either 12 or 36 additional weeks of "peginterferon alfa and ribavirin depending on viral response and prior response status."[7] However, despite a rapid product launch, Incivek was pulled off the market by its manufacturer Vertex due to reported complications ranging from serious skin reactions to death,[7] and sagging sales caused by competition from the more effective and lesser invasive drugs Solvadi and Harvoni produced by Gilead Sciences.[8]

Victrelis® (*boceprevir*), manufactured by Merck, was approved by the FDA in 2011 for "the treatment of chronic hepatitis C genotype 1 infection, in combination with pegainterferon alfa and ribavirin, for the treatment genotype 1 chronic hepatitis C in adult patients with compensated liver disease, including cirrhosis, who are previously untreated or who have failed previous interferon and ribavirin treatment, including prior null responders, partial responders and relapsers… Victrelis must not be used as a monotherapy, and should only be used in combination with peginterferon alfa and ribavirin."[10] It is warned that this drug must not be used by pregnant women or their mates within six months of conception as birth defects and/or fetal death may occur. Treatment begins with four weeks of peginterferon + ribavirin, then Victrelis is added, the duration dependent upon viral load. Adverse reactions include fatigue, anemia, nausea, headache and dysgeusis [taste distortion].[10] In "two phase 3 clinic trials with 1,500 adult patients… two-thirds of the patients receiving Victrelia in combination with pegylated interferon and ribavirin experienced a significantly increased sustained virologic response [HCV not detected 24 weeks post treatment].[11] Victrelis was pulled out of the U. S. market in January 2015, due to the new wave of monotherapy drugs that could be effective without interferon and ribavirin.[12]

Olysio® *(simeprevir)*, manufactured by Janssen-Cilag, was approved by the FDA in 2013, for treatment of adults with HCV with two treatment options: (1) in combination with sofosbuvir for patients genotype 1 without cirrhosis [12 weeks] or with compensated cirrhosis [24 weeks]; (2) in combination with peginterferon alpha and ribavirin for patients genotype 1 or 4 without cirrhosis or with compensated cirrhosis" [12 weeks].[13] Treatment may be extended if warranted by response. Olysio works by blocking a specific protein the HCV needs to replicate. Clinical trials showed an up to an 80 to 90% success rate.[13] Olysio comes in the form of a capsule taken once daily with food. Common side effects include fatigue, headache, nausea, skin rash, and photosensitivity. In extreme cases serious bradycardia [abnormally slow heart rate] has occurred as well as hepatic decompensation and failure [liver].[14]

Viekira Pak® *(ombitasvir, paritaprevir, ritonavir + dasabuvir)*, manufactured byAbbVie, approved by the FDA in 2013, is an all-oral regimen comprised of four medications in two tablets. The ombitasvir-paritaprevir-ritonavir tablet is taken once a day in the morning, and the dasabuvir taken twice a day in the morning and evening. This treatment with ribavirin lasts for 12 weeks for patients with genotype 1a without cirrhosis, and 24 weeks for patients with compensated cirrhosis. Genotype 1b patients, with or without compensated cirrhosis take Viekira Pak for 12 weeks without ribavirin. Reported side effects include fatigue, nausea, pruritus [skin itching / rashes], insomnia and asthenia [physical weakness, lack of energy]. In extreme cases of patients with advanced cirrhosis, hepatic decompensation and failure [liver] have occurred.[15] In clinical trials involving 2,308 participants, 91% to 100% achieved sustained virologic response (SVR).[16]

Solvadi® (*sofobuvir*), manufactured by Gilead Sciences, approved by the FDA in 2013, is a once daily tablet taken in combination with pegylated interferon and/or ribavirin to treat HCV genotypes 1,2,3 and 4. For genotypes 1 and 4, Solvadi is administered with peginterferon alpha and ribavirin for 12 weeks. Solvadi with ribavirin is administered for 12 weeks for genotype 2, and 24 weeks with genotype 3. There are other treatment variations depending upon factors such as co-infection with HIV, patients who are interferon ineligible, patients awaiting liver transplants, and those with severe renal [kidney] impairment or end stage renal disease. Most common side effects include headache, nausea, fatigue, insomnia and anemia. Extreme adverse reactions of symptomatic bradycardia [slow heart rate] have been reported from patients with heart problems or those who are taking beta blockers.[17] In clinical trials Sovadi was shown to be effective in patients not able to tolerate an "interferon-based treatment regimen and in participants with liver cancer awaiting liver transplantation."[18]

Harvoni® (*sofobuvir + ledipasvir*), marketed by Gilead Sciences and approved by the FDA in 2014, was the first is a one-a-day pill used to treat Hepatitis C for genotypes 1, 4, 5, and 6. For genotype 1 patients who are treatment-naïve without cirrhosis or compensated cirrhosis, and patients who are treatment-experienced without cirrhosis, treatment is one Harvoni tablet daily with or without food for 12 weeks. Genotype 1 patients who are treatment-experienced with compensated cirrhosis, take one Harvoni tablet daily for 24 weeks. Patients with genotype 1 who are treatment-naïve or treatment-experienced with decompensated cirrhosis take one Harvoni tablet daily with ribavirin for 12 weeks. Patients with genotypes 1 or 4 who are treatment-naïve or treatment-experienced liver transplant recipients without cirrhosis, or with compensated cirrhosis take one Harvoni tablet daily with ribavirin for 12 weeks. And, patients with genotypes 4, 5 or 6 who are treatment-naïve or treatment-experienced without cirrhosis, or with compensated cirrhosis take one Harvoni tablet daily 12 weeks.[19] Harvoni's efficacy was evaluated in three clinical trials with 1,518 treatment-naïve patients, and patients who had not responded to previous treatment (treatment-experienced). Among treatment-naïve participants, 94% of those who received Harvoni for eight weeks, and 96% of those who received Harvoni for 12 weeks achieved SVR. In another trial, 94% of treatment-experienced participants of those who received Harvoni for 12 weeks, and 99% of those who received Harvoni for 24 weeks achieved SVR.[20] Reported side effects include fatigue, headache and asthenia (physical weakness). Patients are warned not to use Harvoni with beta blockers, St. John's Wort, or amiodarone as bradycardia [slow heartbeat] may occur.[19]

Technivie® (*ombitasvir, paritaprevir + ritonavir*), manufactured by AbbVie, was approved by the FDA in 2015, for treatment of chronic HCV patients with genotype 4 without cirrhosis. Treatment-naïve patients take two tablets of Technvie with or without ribavirin in the morning for 12 weeks. No interferon is necessary.[20] The safety and effectiveness of Technivie was evaluated in a clinical trial of 135 participants with chronic HCV genotype 4 infections; 91 received Technivie + ribavirin, and 44 received just Technivie daily for 12 weeks. Sustained virologic response (SVR) was present in 100% of the participants 12 weeks following the end of treatment. The three drugs in Technivie are also present in Viekira Pak, also produced by AbbVie.[21] Side effects reported include asthenia (physical weakness, lack of energy), fatigue, nausea and insomnia. Some patients with advanced cirrhosis have reported hepatic decompensation and hepatic failure (liver), including liver transplantation or even death.[22]

Daklinza® (*daclatasvir*), manufactured by Bristol-Myers Squibb and approved by the FDA in 2015, has been proven to safely and effectively treat HCV genotypes 1 and 3 without co-administration of ribavirin or interferon, though in some cases ribavirin is indicated.[23] In a clinical trial of 152 treatment-naïve and treatment-experienced participants with HCV genotype 3, Daklinza + sofosbuvir was administered once daily for 12 weeks. HCV was undetected in 98% of the treatment-naïve participants with no cirrhosis, and in 58% of the treatment-naïve participants with cirrhosis, 12 weeks after finishing treatment. Reported side effects include nausea, anemia, fatigue and headache. In some cases when Daklinza was administered with other drugs, slowing of the heart rate (symptomatic bradycardia) has been reported, including situations where pacemaker intervention was required.[24]

Zepatier® (*elbasvir + grazoprevir*) manufacturer by Merck, was approved by the FDA in 2016, for treatment of patients infected by HCV genotypes 1 and 4, either with or without cirrhosis. Treatment criteria are exact, depending upon whether the patient is treatment-naïve, or experienced with prior interferon treatment. In general, treatment consist of one Zepatier tablet a day, with or without ribavirin, for 12 to 16 weeks.[25] In a clinical trial of 1,373 participants with chronic HCV genotype 1 or 4 infections, with or without cirrhosis, one tablet of Zepatier without or without ribavirin was given daily for 12 to 16 weeks. SVR rates 12 weeks following treatment were 94% to 97% for genotype 1 participants and 97-100% for genotype 4 participants across all test groups.[26] Reported side effects include fatigue, headache, nausea and anemia. The product label warns Zapatier should not be given to patients with moderate or severe liver impairment.[25,26]

Epclusa® (*sofobuvir + velpatasvir*) manufactured by Gilead Sciences is the newest HCV daily dose tablet, approved by the FDA in 2016 to treat HCV genotypes 1, 2, 3 ,4, 5 and 6. For patients without cirrhosis or with compensated cirrhosis, one tablet is taken daily for 12 weeks. For patients with decompensated (moderate to severe) cirrhosis, one tablet is taken daily with ribavirin for 12 weeks.[27] The effectiveness of Epclusa was evaluated in three Phase III clinical trials of 1,558 participants without cirrhosis, or with compensated cirrhosis. Results showed 95-99% had undetectable HCV/RNA twelve weeks after finishing the prescribed 12 weeks of taking daily Epclusa tablets. In another clinical trial of participants with decompensated cirrhosis, 94% had no detectable levels in the blood twelve weeks after finishing a 12-week regimen of daily doses of Epclusa plus ribavirin.[28] Side effects reported are typically headache, fatigue, anemia, nausea, insomnia and diarrhea. The package label warns of possible bradycardia with co-administration of amidodarone, especially if they are also taking beta blockers.[27]

TRADE NAME	FDA	COMPANY	GENOTYPES	TYPICAL TREATMENT
Pegagsys® + Copegus®	2002 2002	Genetech Genetech	1,2,3,4 1,2,3,4	Injections 6 to 12 months + Daily tablet
Incivek®*	2011	Vertex	1	Tablets/interferon/ribavirin, 12-48 weeks
Victrelis®*	2011	Merck	1	Tablets/interferon/ribavirin, 12-36 weeks
Olysio®	2013	Janssen-Cilag	1,4	Daily tablet, 24 weeks
Viekira Pak®	2013	AbbVie	1	4 Daily tablets, 12 to 24 weeks
Sovaldi®	2013	Gilead	1,2,3,4	Daily tablet + ribavirin, 12 weeks
Harvoni®	2014	Gilead	1,4,5,6	Daily tablet, 8 to 24 weeks
Technivie®	2015	AbbVie	4	2 Daily tablets + ribavirin, 12 weeks
Daklinza®	2015	Bristol-Meyers Squibb	1,3	Daily tablet w/sofosbuvir, w/wo ribavirin, 12 week
Zepatier®	2016	Merck	1,4	Daily tablet, 12 weeks
Epclusa®	2016	Gilead	1,2,3,4,5,6	Daily tablet w/wo ribavirin 12 weeks
* Discontinued due to market competition by newer more effective drugs.				

Reading the encapsulated descriptions above, you see that most of these modern drugs have a similar set of side effects. When you read through this book you will see many real descriptions of Harvoni patients describing their side effects which will probably be similar to the range of side effects you can expect to experience while taking Harvoni or any other these other drugs: Epclusa, Zapatier, Daklinza, Technivie or Solvadi. The addition of ribavirin may increase or decrease your side effects, or produce others. The table above summarizes the information in this chapter, including: brand name of drug, year approved by the FDA, drug manufacturer or distributor, HCV genotypes on which the drug has been found to be effective, and the typical length and type of treatment, which the drug has been found to be effective, and the typical length and type of treatment.

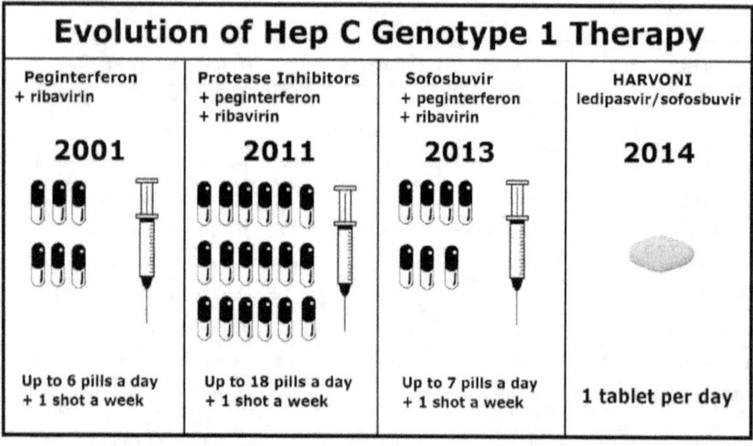

Since the advent of these new "miracle" substances, pharmaceutical companies have recently been fast-tracking new labeled products into the marketplace which hold the promise to cure the hundreds of millions of people worldwide suffering from acute and chronic Hep C. Many others are unaware they have the disease while it slowly grows inside and can lead to liver cancer and other diseases responsible for over 700,000 deaths each year.[31,33,34] The beauty of these new drugs is the ease of treatment – one pill a day instead of a complex regimen of pills and shots. The graphic below provides a dramatic snapshot of the advancement of the Harvoni regimen over previous treatments. This class of HCV drugs has been one of the most rapidly developed and profitable in the history of modern pharmaceuticals. The good news is these drugs are having amazing success (95% - 100% in some cases) at reducing HCV/RNA down to undetectable levels. As newer more effective drugs enter the market, manufacturers withdraw the older less effective ones.

But, the price tag is still extraordinarily high, as much as $1,100 a pill for Harvoni which, over the course of a 12-week treatment, adds up to $92,400 – a figure not many people can afford. My next challenge was to find out if I could get approved under my insurance plan to take Harvoni, the drug my doctor said had the best chance of reducing my HCV to undetectable levels.

GETTING APPROVED

Harvoni is an expensive drug. The sticker price for a 12-week treatment costs about $94,000, nearly a $1,100 a day. Insurance companies started scrambling to coordinate payment options with prescribing physicians. Hard choices had to be made about who would get the drug and who would not. I really don't know much about the politics of all this, as who is able to receive Harvoni, and who isn't, was often a mystery based on a complicated algorithm that was specific to location, the doctors and the type of insurance. Was the criteria based on the age and gender of the patient along with the extent of the liver damage? No one seemed to know for sure.

I found another gastroenterologist in our new town and found her to be much more caring and compassionate than my previous doctor. She had my blood sample drawn and again found that my AST, ALT and ALP levels were extremely elevated. She then ordered a more focused blood test to measure HCV/RNA, which would indicate the extent of my Hep C viral load.[1,2]

Liver damage is assessed by the statistical measure of HCV/RNA levels in the blood. HCV stands for Hepatitis C Virus, and RNA stands for ribonucleic acid, which carries genetic information used in synthesizing proteins. In the blood test, the amount of the Hep C virus per given volume of blood (usually 1 cubic centimeter, or cc) is known as the viral load. The viral load of the Hep C virus can range from being undetected to hundreds of millions. Once the viral load drops to the undetected level six months after treatment, "long term cure is highly probable."[1]

As time progressed, my viral load had increased to over 4.5 million and rising, making me a good candidate to receive Harvoni treatment. Unfortunately, the damage to my liver was not severe enough, as it was assessed to only be in Stage 2 Hepatitis where I needed Stage 3 or 4 to jump to the front of the line to qualify.

When someone first contracts Hepatitis C, they enter the acute phase which may or may not be accompanied with physical symptoms of abdominal pain, loss of appetite, dark urine, fatigue, fever, gray-colored stools, joint pain, nausea, vomiting, a yellowing of the skin and whites of the eyes. If the body cannot fight off the disease in six months, it progresses to the chronic phase where the virus lives in the body. This can go undetected for many years until a doctor recognizes high levels of liver enzymes during a routine blood test. As the disease progress, it passes through four stages:

Stage 0 – no fibrosis, or scarring.
Stage 1 – mild inflammation but little or no scarring.
Stage 2 – mild to moderate fibrosis.
Stage 3 – bridging fibrosis spreading throughout the liver.
Stage 4 – severe scarring, or cirrhosis.

Left untreated, cirrhosis can progress until the liver loses all function, resulting in death."[3,4]

The look on the face of my gastroenterologist pained me as much as the pain I felt myself. She said: "Don't worry, we are going to submit your test results again and will keep trying until you get approved."

It was ironic that I almost had to get cirrhosis before I could get the drug that prevented the cirrhosis! This news was devastating to me as I had been feeling worse and worse every day. It was hard to get out of bed to clean the house or run simple errands. Spending a day with my granddaughter exhausted me so, I had to sleep the entire next day to recover. Sometimes I would leave the house, get in my car, and forget how to get to a place I had been a hundred times. I would sit with the car running, trying to remember, eventually resorting to the GPS on my phone to lead me there.

It was like my brain was in a constant fog. I couldn't understand the simplest things people said to me. I would start to say something and forget the words I was trying to say. It was like my mind went totally blank. I avoided people because I didn't want to feel embarrassed in conversation. I gave up reading because I lost the continuity of what was going on in the book. My attention span reminded me of what I had observed of my father-in-law as he was dying of Alzheimer's. I did not know it at the time, but this is a common condition with Hep C sufferers known as Hepatic Encephalopathy:

"If liver cells are damaged, certain substances that are normally cleansed from the blood by the healthy liver are not removed (ammonia mainly, and other toxins). A patient with chronic hepatic encephalopathy may develop progressive loss of memory, disorientation, untidiness, and muscular tremors, leading to a form of chronic dementia. The ingestion of protein invariably aggravates these symptoms."[5]

This was terribly frustrating and kept me in a constant bad mood. I found myself drinking to kill the pain. Drinking made me sociable and feel somewhat normal, allowing me to forget I had this disease, until I went to bed and the alcohol wore off. Then, I was reacquainted with my old nemesis: *The Dragon.* My body would itch and be on fire and I would wake up with no feeling in my fingers, the beginnings of neuropathy.

When your liver malfunctions, the malaise spreads throughout your body, diminishing normal functioning. The whites of my eyes were jaundiced and bloodshot, requiring me to use eye drops frequently and wear sunglasses when I went out in public. I often fought off double vision. My skin itched so often I feared I would scratch my skin off down to the blood. I lost my appetite and felt full on just a few bites of food. I began to experience digestive problems evidenced by profuse flatulence. It was like a war was going on inside my organs. These are all reported symptoms of people who have advancing liver damage due to Hepatitis C.

At that point, my only option was to find a way to come up with $94,000. But, I didn't want to give up. Descriptions about all sorts of new ways to get HCV drugs started appearing online. People in the Hep C chat rooms were talking about people they knew who had gone to India where generic Harvoni was available for $9 a pill, a full 12-week treatment costing under a thousand dollars. Or going to other countries in Europe in Asia on a 'Hep C treatment holiday,' as did Phillip Smith, who was confronted by a situation typical of many Hep C patients:

"My Affordable Care Act insurance plan would, for a time cover the treatment – but only if my liver was already diseased. In other words, I had to let the disease progress to the point that it actually threatened my life before the insurance company would pay to treat the disease… There was another problem. Because I had a low-premium high-deductible health insurance plan, even if my insurance company paid for the drugs, I still faced $6,000 in out-of-pocket costs."[6]

Smith did some research online and found that Gilead, makers of Harvoni, had entered into an agreement with overseas drug manufacturers to produce generic versions of the Harvoni and Solvaldi for sale in developing countries with severe HCV problems in the population. In India, Smith found several vendors willing to sell a full 12-week treatment regimen of generic Harvoni (Hepcinat LP) for $1500 and selected a company called Care Exim (http://www.buygenericdrugonline.com/search.html?ss=Hepcinat%20LP) which did not require a doctor's prescription. Care Exim did not accept credit cards, so Smith took a chance and sent a bank wire transfer.

"I paid my money and took my chances. The package arrived in nine days, untouched by customs. There were indeed three bottle of pills labeled as Hepcinat LP manufactured by Natco, with seals and even a folded paper insert with all the drug information on it. I took the pills for 83 days (saving one for possible testing just in case), waited a couple weeks, then went to my doctor and had my blood drawn. The following

week, he reported that my hepatitis C viral load was now zero."[6]

Smith's case is a bold example of how Hep C can motivate a person to take extreme measures to feel better. However, people living in rich Western countries going overseas for low-cost medical treatment is not new. Elderly Americans on fixed incomes have been flocking to Canada for years to buy prescription medicine, either in person across the border or via online pharmacies who ship to the U.S. after submitting a legitimate physician's prescription.

Like anything else in life, going overseas to receive medical treatment or to purchase drugs, requires vigilance as unscrupulous purveyors are out there eager to steal your money. "Shoppers risk their health when they buy from pharmacies they don't know," says Mark Turnage, CEO of Denver-based OpSec, a firm that provides anti-counterfeiting services to over 300 brands and 50 governments. "About 10% of pharmaceuticals are counterfeit, and that number rises when they're sold online."

Two others firms that verify the legitimacy of online pharmacies are LegitScript.com and PharmacyChecker.com, which also provide links to purchase pharmaceuticals.[7] Patients requiring cheap medicine, joint replacement surgery, or desiring plastic surgery, can find qualified doctors in Mexico, Spain or other countries eager to take U. S. dollars.[8] These services can be arranged through the Medical Tourism Association "a membership based international non-profit trade association for the medical tourism and global healthcare industry made up of the top international hospitals, healthcare providers, medical travel facilitators, insurance companies, and other affiliated companies and members with the common goal of promoting the highest level of quality of healthcare to patients in a global environment." (medicaltourismassociation.com)

Another company currently assembling a network of doctors and foreign hospitals willing to prescribe drugs to U. S. patients is Health Flight Solutions in Orlando, Florida. CEO Anuja Agrawal says her company "is working with the generic drug manufacturers to verify hospitals in her network aren't getting counterfeit drugs."[9]

But, many Americans are unaware of the Federal Food and Drug Cosmetic Act [*21 U. S. Code 301*, amended 2002] which prohibits importation of pharmaceuticals without approval of the FDA. So, ordering Hep C drugs from foreign companies is not without legal risk, in addition to not getting the authentic mixture of the HCV fighting compounds produced by Gilead, AbbVie, Bristol-Myers Squibb, Merck and other U. S. companies who are beginning to respond to the pressures being applied by sick patients who eagerly desire treatment.

Gilead has offered a co-pay coupon that provides discounts up to 25% off the catalogue price for patients with commercial insurance, or cash-pay patients, for non-reimbursable prescriptions.[10] A similar program has been offered by AbbVie for Viekira Pak[11]. New discount programs may appear at any time, so check the drug manufacturers' websites listed in the Appendices for the latest promotions on HCV fighting drugs.

In March 2016, Gilead Sciences was court ordered to pay Merck $200 million in damages for infringing on its patents for sofosbuvir, a key ingredient in both Solvadi and

Harvoni. In 2015, Gilead worldwide sales for its two HCV fighting drugs reached $19.1 billion, accounting for 2/3s of the company's revenue. Total U. S. sales for Solvadi and Harvoni through 2015 amounted to a staggering $23.1 billion.

Despite paying $11 billion in 2011 to Pharmasset for rights to the then experimental drug sofosbuvir, and subsequent developments and testing costs, Harvoni and Solvadi have been two of the most successful drugs ever launched.[12] And, with price tags upwards of $90,000 for a 12-week treatment, HCV patients, doctors and insurance companies have started to rally around promoting legislation that would mandate prices down to reasonable levels.[13]

Insurance companies are only allowing the expensive Hep C drugs to patients with advanced or severe liver disease, denying claims to 80% of those who apply. Three common policies are used by insurance companies to limit access. First, patients need to be diagnosed with either stage 3 or stage 4 liver disease, the rationale being people can live for 30 years or more with HCV and only the sickest need immediate treatment.[14]

Second, patients are required to take urine tests that attest to their sobriety from drugs and alcohol for usually three consecutive months; if a person is using drugs or drinking heavily they are voluntarily harming themselves. Third, the patient's condition must be assessed by, and prescription written by not just any licensed physician, but a liver specialist – a problem in many areas without enough specialists to serve the population.[15]

The primary justification for the high cost of HCV drugs is that they can cure HCV and thus save the insurance companies the cost of a liver transplant that can run $250,000.

However, this rationale does little to assuage the sting of the high cost of treatment for many people whose medical care is provided by the government. Hepatitis C disproportionately effects lower-income people who are on Medicaid and people who are incarcerated. Although HCV can be contracted through blood transfusions, needle sticks to healthcare workers, piercings, tattoos, or through any type of blood-to-blood contact, the unspoken opinion of many is that it is the province of drug users. "Stigma plays a huge role in this," says Ryan Clary, executive director of the National Viral Hepatitis Roundtable, an advocacy group. "If it were another disease that didn't have the same sort of stigma, I don't think we'd have the same conversation."[13]

The viral hepatitis epidemic (A, B and C) is reminiscent of the HIV/AIDS situation that occurred in the United States back in the 1980s. All are blood-born viruses which can remain undetected for many years. Healthcare workers on the front lines see parallels with the "early years of the AIDs epidemic, when a combination of misinformation and unwillingness to candidly address stigmatized behaviours and social inequalities led to widespread failure to formulate a cohesive public health response."[16] With new drugs now available such as Solvadi, Harvoni, Zepatier, Danzlinza and Epclusa, control and elimination of the hepatitis C virus is a real possibility, just as polio was virtually eradicated in the United States in 1979.[17]

Back to my story…

I saw my doctor a couple months later. She ran some more blood tests and found that my liver enzymes and viral load continued to climb. In addition, she requested a new test that would assess the actual damage to my liver. It was called Magnetic Resonance Elastography (MRE).[18] I lay back on a table while the technician ran a device over my skin above my liver. It was much like the Sonogram I had when I was pregnant, but instead of images of my new baby, the screen showed pictures of my liver. While the blood and MRE test results were being compiled, my doctor suggested that I call Gilead, the makers of Harvoni directly to see if there was any kind of program available for which I might qualify.

"We'll keep trying," my doctor said. We both had tears in our eyes when we hugged.

I left the sanctuary of her office and returned to the outside world that was growing increasingly unfriendly. I had seriously been thinking about suicide and ways I might accomplish it with the least discomfort. I thought about tying a rope around my neck, tying it to the upstairs banister, and jumping down toward the foyer. Or, overdosing on pills. I felt so depressed I didn't care how my death would affect others. In short, I was a mess. One night I slipped, drank a couple glasses of wine and thought I was going to die. My mate had to call EMS to take me to the emergency room where they gave me an IV overnight and ran some more tests.

A couple days later I remembered what my doctor had said about contacting the drug manufacturer directly and thought I'd give it a shot. I went online and looked up the Harvoni helpline number at Gilead (855-769-7284, M-F 9 a.m to 8 p.m. EST). The representative answered right away after a couple of prompts and seemed most concerned and friendly as I explained my condition. She then asked me a series of screening questions and told me I needed to assemble all my paperwork and send for their review. They wanted blood and other tests results, a letter from my doctor and a personal letter explaining my situation. She gave me the address where to send and said it would take several weeks for a reply. I thanked them and hung up, exhausted from the call, putting assembly of the documents off until the next day.

I was on my second cup of coffee trying to focus my mind enough to start compiling what the Gilead representative had wanted when my phone rang. My test results were in and I had to go see my doctor.

"Valerie I have good news and bad news," she said, entering the examining room, nicely dressed with a smile.

"What's the good news?" I asked eagerly.

"Your tests came back and I think I can finally get you approved!"

"Okay," I said, not jumping for joy. "What's the bad news?"

"The MRE shows fibrosis on your liver. But, not to worry because I don't think you have cirrhosis. We will check that when you are done with treatment. Everything's going to be fine."

My mind was too foggy to immediately comprehend what was happening. I would be approved. I would get the Harvoni which could drop my viral loads down to an undetectable level. I would not die right away by Hepatitis C, or by my own hand. I would be able to live a near normal life.

"But, you have to work with me," my doctor insisted. "You have to stop drinking and change your diet. Harvoni works best when you respect the treatment and contribute with life style changes."

I agreed wholeheartedly. Finally, a cure was possible and I was motivated to do everything I could to help maximize the treatment's potential. I was told to stop taking all the various vitamins and herbs I had been buying in health food stores and on line. I was to lay off red meat, start exercising and drink lots of water. I bought a juicer and started making concoctions of juice from beets, kale, lemons, celery, apples, ginger, and other fresh fruits and vegetables. I limited my animal protein to fish and chicken.

I also mixed up a new powered shake called Soylent with chocolate whey protein. Soylent is a product developed by several entrepreneurs in San Francisco who sought to find a food formula that perfectly met the nutritional needs of the human body. Their story is quite interesting and the food product is great. My body loves it. Read all about at www.soylent.com.

A couple days later my pharmacist called. My doctor had gotten approval, he had placed the order and my first bottle of Harvoni would arrive the next week!

PRE-TREATMENT PREPARATION

The days leading up to beginning the Harvoni treatment were both exciting and nerve-racking. I didn't have the energy to go to the gym and about all I could manage was keeping the house clean and walking the dog. A couple times a week I had the joy of picking my granddaughter up from school and playing with her the four exhausting hours before her mother got off work. Then I would hit the sheets and sleep until mid-morning the next day.

I had changed my diet completely and was juicing like crazy and drinking lots of water. I read articles online and bought several books, one of the best being *The Hepatitis C Cookbook* by Heather Jeanne. The book is full of tasty recipes and some excellent pointers about what and how to eat to make it easy on your liver. Jeanne compares the filtering functions of the liver to a filter on an air-conditioner:

"...it gets dirty. The more you run your air conditioner, the more dirt its filter collects. If you do not clean or replace the filter, side effects begin to occur: the machinery becomes less efficient and works harder to perform, your electric bill increases, fewer germs and allergens will be removed, and your air will remain contaminated."[1]

This is why a proper diet and drinking plenty of pure water is so important during treatment. In addition, Jeanne offers these helpful tips to help your liver:

- Use fresh products and whole foods.
- Read the labels to make sure you know what you are getting.
- Grow fruits and vegetables yourself if you have the space and time.
- Eat small easy to digest meals, and your main meal between noon and 2:00 p.m.
- Don't eat meat and dairy in the same meal, like chicken Alfredo.
- Don't use cast iron cookware as it imparts iron into the food.
- Broccoli, Brussels sprouts, cabbage and cauliflower promote liver proteins.
- Steam rather than boil or overcook vegetables.
- Use low or reduced fat dairy products.
- Don't use artificial sweeteners. Use raw organic sugar or honey.
- When using a fat, choose olive oil, unsalted butter or ghee.
- Avoid all alcoholic products and soft drinks.

A more recent article published on the Hepatitis Central website, added five anti-inflammatory guidelines condensed from health research. Implementing these principles into your diet will lessen the stress on your damaged liver and help promote more rapid healing.

1. *"**Eat good fat** – cold water fish like salmon, trout, mackerel, tuna and sardines; avocados, extra-virgin olive oil, coconut oil, flax seeds, hemp seeds, nuts, and expeller-pressed, organic canola oil.*

2. ***Fiber** – Brown rice, quinoa, barley, oatmeal, okra, eggplant, apples, avocado, banana, berries, figs, artichokes, peas, acorn squash, black beans, lima beans, lentils, almonds and chia seeds.*

3. ***Fruit and Veggies** – Spinach, dandelion greens, kale, carrots, celery, squash, berries, oranges, lemons, melons, peppers, asparagus, green beans, tomatoes, bok choy, onions, bananas, apples, pears, arugula, yams, beets, pineapple, collards and cherries.*

4. ***Antioxidants** – Brightly colored produce, green leafy vegetables, green tea, turmeric, ginger, tart cherries, garlic, dark chocolate, tomatoes, citrus fruit, broccoli, nuts, chili peppers, beets and grapes.*

5. ***Skip These Foods** – Fast food, deep-fried food, pastries, vegetable shortenings, margarines, crackers, cakes, cookies, palm oil, poultry skin, fatty dairy foods, fatty pork or beef, non-dairy creamer, artificial sweeteners, soda, sugar, white bread, alcohol, MSG and chips".*[2]

After getting a good grip on what my diet should be like, I started doing research online about Harvoni and read everything I could possibly find, from detailed scientific articles and information posted on the Gilead website, to chat rooms where the thoughts, opinions and experiences of others who were at different stages in the Harvoni treatment program. I also visited other chat rooms where other Hep C treatment drugs were being discussed to provide me with as full a body of knowledge as possible. We all had the common bound of inflammation in our livers and were fighting to stay alive until we could complete treatment. I was also able to read about the experiences of others weeks further down the line, who were expressing side effects, anxieties, elations, reduced physical symptoms and increasing energy. A list of some of the best Harvoni and Hep C discussion groups, chat rooms and message boards are listed in the reference section at the end of the book. Here are some comments pre-treatment several of my Hep C friends posted online [edited and anonymized, of course].

"I have had Hep C for 28 years, am 57- years-old and will be starting in two weeks. I hope and pray it works for me."

"My Harvoni approval came through and I should get the call any day my pills are in at the pharmacy. I tried interferon/ribavirin years ago and it didn't work. Your words are encouraging."

"I have mild cirrhosis and am genotype 1. High hopes the Harvoni will do the trick. Did not want to try interferon and waited for over 15 years."

"I contracted Hep C through a blood transfusion. After a friend of mine died from a Hep C treatment, I was scared to try anything. I am so glad Harvoni came along. I'm on my

first week and the side effects are nothing compared to what I had been living with. I work long hours at a stressful job and can't afford to be down."

"The horror stories I have heard about interferon have kept me away from treatment until now. Harvoni sounds like a miracle cure and I am looking into getting treatment."

"My father died of liver cancer and it was a horrible painful way to go. Since I found out I had Hep C, I have been waiting for the low impact drugs to develop. I tried the interferon / ribavirin thing and it made me so sick, daily pills plus three injections a week. I have a friend who works in HCV research and told me about new drugs in clinical trials. At last, Harvoni!"

"I still am having side effects from the interferon treatment I took a decade ago. My liver was so shot I had to have a transplant. I feel better, but still have the Hep C. I fear Harvoni won't work, but it looks like my only chance at having a decent life."

"It's a little scary knowing that tomorrow I start on Harvoni. I don't know what to expect. I still have painful memories of the interferon / ribavirin I did twelve years ago. It was so bad I had to drop out of treatment. I hear Harvoni is quicker with hardly any side effects. We will see, but I am hopeful."

It was gratifying to read that I was not alone in my fears, worries and concerns, and that there was a whole community of people out there I could communicate with, and share the truth about my upcoming experience. This gave me a great deal of comfort and confidence that I was doing the right thing. I was glad I didn't give in years ago and take the interferon treatment and that waiting for Harvoni might be one of the best decisions I ever made.

The next day I went to my last pre-treatment doctor's appointment, and she assured me everything would be all right. The pharmacist then arrived for a consultation with my first bottle of Harvoni. I chatted with the pharmacist for almost an hour. She was very thorough and kind and told me I was the most informed patient she had, and praised me for what I had learned from all the research I had done on the internet. She wished others would do the same as it would make her job easier and help alleviate the fears and worries other patients expressed to her.

We discussed the side effects including fatigue which typically appeared two days after the first dose, but I had been living in a state of fatigue for so long anything seemed like it would be an improvement. She said I would probably get headaches and to only take Tylenol – not aspirin, Advil or anything else. She also said for me to drink at least 64 ounces of pure water every day as it would help ward off the headaches and facilitate flushing the virus out of my system.

I told her that I joined an online Harvoni support group and noticed other people talking about many other side effects such as ulcers in the mouth, anxiety attacks, ringing in the ears, irritability, depression, nose bleeds, extreme muscle and joint aches and lack of sleep. Again she reiterated not only had I done my research but was genuinely excited that there was such support group on Facebook. The doctor said she would love to post hard printed copies of post-treatment blood results showing undetected HCV/RNA in her office of all patients cured of Hep C to encourage others, marking out their names to protect their anonymity.

I was given a sheet of all future doctor's appointments and lab work to be done for the next 12 weeks including my 3 and 6 month labs. She also agreed with my disappointment that I had to wait until I was at stage 3/4 of my disease, and explained that I could live a long life when my HCV was cured. The pharmacist then gave me my first of three bottles of Harvoni, saying the next two bottles would be shipped to my home via FedEx.

THE FIRST WEEK:
Fears and Worries

In my hand I held over $30,000 worth of medication at current posted prices. After all those years of waiting and worrying, I finally was going to begin to fight the fire-breathing dragon of HCV.

This may sound strange, but my primary worries at that moment were that Harvoni would not live up to its promises, that my Hep C would not be reduced to undetectable levels, and that I would be stuck feeling horrible forever. It was like I was trying to climb a mountain while dragging a sack full of rocks. I wanted to jettison the sack and be unencumbered by the fatigue, brain fog, depression and other symptoms all those afflicted with HCV suffer, to one degree or another. I was trusting Harvoni to be my dragon slayer.

I took my first pill around noon on May 10, 2016, and that night started to feel effects similar to a double dose of the antibiotic Cipro. I felt jittery and could feel something going on in my stomach like a fight or something. I became hypersensitive to noise, couldn't even listen to the TV and needed complete silence. My mate, who observed me closely through the first couple days, asked if he could do anything, but all I wanted to do was lay down and focus on what effects the Harvoni was creating inside my body.

I may have exacerbated the symptoms through my desire of wanting the drug to attack and vanquish the disease.

But, it did actually feel like the battle lines had been drawn and the sleeping dragon that had its way with me for four decades was being awakened from its cave. Not bad for my first dose, I thought, and fell asleep easily knowing the Harvoni was beginning to effect a cure. I slept most of that first day and night, getting up to use the rest room, have a simple liquid meal, and drink plenty of water.

I decided I would take the Harvoni first thing each morning, so I set the next day's tablet next to a fresh bottle of water on my night stand so it would be ready when I awoke and I wouldn't forget. This may seem silly, but coming from a Catholic school background, I regarded the Harvoni experience as a kind of ritual that had to be observed and respected. I felt this attitude would positively affect the cure.

I awoke about 7 a.m. on the second day, stretched, patted my cat, and picked up the Harvoni tablet from the night stand, and downed it with a full 16 oz. bottle of pure water. I felt remarkably rested and upbeat, confident that I was on my way to a healthy new life, soon to be free of the virus in 83 more days, maybe even sooner. I wrote an initial entry in my daily journal I had started a couple weeks before. The journal entries of my Harvoni experience form the backbone of this book.

I was curious about how others felt as they approached day one of *The Harvoni Experience* and went online. Here are two of the thoughts and feelings they shared.

"I started my eight weeks of treatment yesterday, and it was a very emotional experience thinking a cure for Hep C is

possible. I had a slight headache, but that could be from the anxiety. I take it before bed time so I can sleep through the side effects (if any?)."

"I'm male, 59-years-old, have had diabetes for a decade and Hep C for about 28 years. I took my first dose of Harvoni last night, slept well, but had a slight headache when I woke up. When I started moving around I felt the fatigue coming on and a lack of mental clarity. This could be from the drug beginning to take effect in my system. I need to remember not to allow myself to get frustrated or impatient and give myself time to heal."

I felt fine throughout that entire second day, the third day and the rest of the week with no recognizable symptoms. If anything, the Harvoni seemed to give me a boost of energy that jump started my mornings. Maybe I was buoyed by my enthusiasm or positive attitude, but my fears and worries seemed to dissipate as I went downstairs and prepared a pitcher of a special detox juice mix I had started a couple weeks before. I had gone to the market for fresh produce I chopped and stuffed into the whirling blades of my juicer: beets, carrots, cucumber, celery, lemons, apples, ginger, kale, beet greens, dandelion leaves and turmeric. I poured a tall glass, put the rest of the juice in the refrigerator, and took it to my computer to visit a Harvoni website and see how my friends shared their views on beginning the Harvoni experience.

"I take Harvoni first thing in the morning on an empty stomach as my doctor said it absorbs into the blood stream

quicker. I tried the Incivek with interferon and ribavirin and it didn't work. My liver is in stage 1 fibrosis. To help me sleep I sometimes take Zoloft my doc says is okay."

"I starting taking Harvoni first thing in the morning, but after the third day began experiencing headaches and fatigue. I now take it at night so I can sleep through the side effects. I wake up clearer with more energy."

"I have Type-2 diabetes and stage 2 cirrhosis and am taking Harvoni with ribavirin. It's my third day and I feel nauseated, fatigued and have headaches. I'm thinking my side effects are worse because my liver disease is worse than some of the others who have posted in this room. It may get tough, but anything is worth eradicating this the HCV."

"Fatigue hit me the first day and continues. I want to go back to bed but if this is as bad as it gets I am way ahead of the game."

"I started four days ago and have a slight case of insomnia. While some people report fatigue, the Harvoni seems to affect me the opposite way. Others have reported that too. I wonder if it has something to do with the genotype, body chemistry, what?"

"I'm a diabetic and on my fourth day. The first day was tiring and headaches woke me up the first couple nights. But the side effects seem to have gone away. I hope so. There seems to be no conflict between the Harvoni and my insulin."

"Had my fourth pill today. No problems so far. Take it at 7:00 pm. I also do organic protein shakes in the afternoon that gives me some energy during work. I have gone through the interferon, ribavirin years ago. This will be a cake walk compared to that (hopefully)."

"The first few days I felt really hungry and started taking protein drinks in the afternoon. That helped and gave me energy. I tried the interferon years ago and it didn't work and I felt horrible. Hopefully this will be a walk in the park."

"First day I had stomach cramps and nausea which eased off the second day. Next couple days I was fatigued, impatient and snappy. Fifth day headaches and more hunger than usual, so I eat more. Loose bowels and my liver is tender to the touch. I think the Harvoni is working."

"I'm a 58-year-old male, on my 5th day, I wake up early and have lots of energy."

"I am 66 years old and have had Hep C since 1988. My side effects have been very few, just a slight headache here and there during the past 5 days. It may be because I take the Harvoni after a late breakfast and drink lots of water throughout the day. In my preparation I found that 4-5 small meals is easier on the liver than a couple large ones, so I do that. Otherwise life goes on as usual."

"It's been six days since I started Harvoni. I have had headaches, some loss of mental clarity and pains in my knees

and ankles. But, no big deal. It's easier to get out of bed thinking the cure is at hand."

"I'm am feeling horrible and it is just my sixth day. I'm hoping it will get better."

"I started a low salt diet with no red meat before starting Harvoni six days ago which has resulted in weight loss. I am on my 6th day, have good energy but am experiencing some itching, headaches and loose bowels. I have stopped coffee for the caffeine and soft drinks, so I am doing all the right things to facilitate the cure."

As I read over the postings, a couple things occurred to me. First, some people preferred to take the Harvoni in the morning to start their day like I did. Others preferred to take it before bedtime they would sleep through any symptoms that might occur. Some people felt Harvoni gave them a boost of energy while others thought it made them more fatigued.

Secondly, there were many common side effects as mentioned in the Harvoni package insert with varying degrees of severity: headaches, fatigue, nausea, aches and pains.

Third, most of the reported symptoms were minor or manageable, people seemed to take them in stride knowing the treatment would have ancillary side effects, but that the cure was worth the trouble. Only one person said she felt "horrible." This made me wonder about lifestyle variables and if they had any effect on magnifying or reducing side effects. This notion would become clearer as time went on. After the first week, there were a flurry of reports, such as:

"I have been taking Harvoni for 7 days, have been feeling fatigued in the mornings, but it seemed to wear off as the day progressed. I found that if I increased my water intake the symptoms lessened. Thus, I kept a bottle of water next to my bed so I could drink when thirsty. Drinking plenty of water is very important. I am not the only one who has stated this. I make sure I drink water at least 4-5 times a day."

"I am a very active 63-year-old who exercises almost every day in yoga and aerobics classes. Keeping fit seems to give a boost to the Harvoni effects and minimizes any side effects. I don't think I have had to slow down and can work like usual. Exercise and lots of water are key."

"I just finished my first of eight weeks taking Harvoni. I have been experiencing some twitching in my muscles, especially my eyes. I don't know if this is normal, but have not seen others mention it."

Twitching, hungry, thirsty, tired – all of these side effects seem to be lessened with exercise and drinking lots of water. This is not so different than life without Harvoni. Next, a couple of participants weighed in on the drinking alcohol issue.

"I am on day 7 and cannot report any appreciable side effects. I have a family vacation coming up and there is going to be drinking involved. It would be a shame if I couldn't drink a beer or two with my bros for a couple days. I know it's recommended not to drink as it taxes the liver. But, come on, a couple brews??"

"I'm no expert, but I would suggest talking this over with your doctor. Everything I've read said to respect the treatment enough you need to refrain from imbibing alcohol in any form. I feel grateful I have been allotted a chance to become Hep C free and I'm not going to consciously do anything to screw it up. Just say'n..."

I, personally, had sworn off alcohol in any form the week prior and during my course of treatment. I followed this regimen religiously. I had been suffering with Hep C for years and anything I might consciously do that would negatively impact the efficacy of the treatment I removed from my life. But, this comment made me curious and I went online to see what the experts might say. Keywords are essential to getting focused responses from a Google search, so I typed in "alcohol + Harvoni" and found this concise summary statement from a reputable source:

"The answer from several leading organizations is: no. You should not drink alcohol while taking this drug. The HCV Advocate is a nonprofit support group that offers advice for hepatitis C patients. This group recommends that you completely avoid alcohol if you have hepatitis C. This is especially important if you're having drug treatment for the virus. The American Association for the Study of Liver Diseases (AASLD) and the National Institutes of Health (NIH) Consensus statement agree. They both strongly recommend that you avoid drinking alcohol if you have hepatitis C."[1]

On message boards, other Harvoni patients were quite candid in expressing their views about using alcohol during treatment:

"If you have Hep C, drinking booze should be the last thing on your mind."

"My doctor never said I couldn't have one beer. Should I ask him or just go ahead and see how I feel?"

"Why would anyone who has Hep C or any kind of liver disease want to drink alcohol, especially if you have a chance to be cured? It's mind boggling to me."

"My doctor said drinking a couple beers a week is okay and shouldn't cause much damage." [Really now?]

"I've read that drinking can make some of the side effects worse and might neutralize the effects of the Harvoni. Why risk it?"

"I used to like to drink for relaxation and to socialize, but I am not giving in to the urge to drink as I know it can only adversely affect the treatment."

"It's well-documented in the research that alcohol is poisonous to the liver. Why burden the liver any more with drinking when you have Hep C?"

"Though Hep C causes a different kind of damage to the liver than alcohol, they both damage the liver. I am trying to heal my liver, not destroy it."

I decided to choose the scientific view and common sense over any urge I had to consume alcohol while taking Harvoni. I found a glass of bubbly Pellegrino over ice with a slice of lemon did wonders to offset the psychological need to hold a drink in my hand. Plus, it made me feel good through hydrating my body and, I do believe, helped stave off any magnification of symptoms alcohol may have caused.
In short, many of the fears, worries and concerns about what Harvoni would be like we had before we started treatment, seemed to fall to the wayside for most of us once the first tablet made its way into our systems and started fighting the disease. This became clear after the first week of treatment. It was like the anxious fighter going into the ring who is nervous as politician before the Pearly Gates, but once the bell rang, the nerves settled and a calm focused plan of attack took over, leading the warrior to victory.

WEEKS 2 – 4:
Typical Side Effects

After the exhilaration of beginning Harvoni, and the realization that the symptoms after one week were relatively minor, I was settling into a routine I would follow for the entire twelve weeks of treatment. Harvoni tablet with a bottle of pure water upon awakening so the drug could go to work immediately before food, then coffee. I would wait until mid-morning to imbibe a drink of pure natural juices or the Soylent mixed with whey protein powder. Then, walk the dog, go to the gym, chores around the house, grocery shopping, pick up my granddaughter after school, feed her, help her with her homework until her mother came back from work, and so forth, getting to bed early to get a healthy night's rest. I'm 60 years old and glad I was past the years when I had to go to a full-time job. Most of the people I've talked with in Harvoni chat rooms are from the 'baby-boomer' era, though there are younger people and even spry folks in their eighties.

So, all was well in the world, though I did have a battle going on in my body as the Harvoni seemed to move around and attack the virus wherever it was hiding. Some days I could feel the battle going on in the liver. Other days it might be in a joint or a muscle in another part of my body. I was curious about this and did some research on viruses.

The body's immune system is the enemy of viruses. To survive and infect the organism, viruses must reproduce faster than the immune system can defeat them. Some viruses, including Herpes and Shingles, hide in the body and lay dormant for years until conditions become favorable for infection. Most viruses, such as the rhinoviruses which cause the common cold, are not that clever and are usually attacked and wiped out by the immune system in a week or so. These viruses mutate slowly over time, copying and recopying their DNA.

Hepatitis C belongs to the RNA class of viruses which are much sneakier and become surrounded within the membrane of infected cells. This masks the identity of HCV and becomes virtually invisible to the immune system.[1] And, it wasn't until recently that new drugs, such as Harvoni, were able to detect and attack the Hep C virus. Thus, it was surprising to me when I got a horrible pain in a back right molar during dinner out with my mate. My teeth are in excellent shape, so I thought maybe a crown had worked itself loose, exposing the nerve, it was so painful. But I couldn't find it. Maybe I had developed a cavity?

The next morning the pain was still there, but it had moved around in my gums. All my teeth seemed to hurt. I also had a small ulcer inside my left cheek. Then, the pain went away, but returned a couple days later. I booked an appointment with my dentist ASAP. She examined me and found nothing out of sorts. I got the impression that maybe she thought I was a hypochondriac, but her calm manner assured me everything would be all right. Could it be that the Hep C virus was hiding in damaged cells from dental work done years ago? I had required several implants, but before they could insert the posts I had liquefied bone injected into my gums to build up the foundation. Perhaps the sneaky virus had also taken up residence there, only to be later detected and eradicated by the Harvoni. No one seemed to know.

Perhaps this is something that could be studied by hepatologists doing advanced research on Hep C.
Lying in bed on the night of day ten, I felt like a huge battle was going on inside my stomach. On day eleven, I felt super fatigued. If I had a job I would have called in and said I had an eye problem ("I can't see getting out of the bed today!").

On day twelve, I was besieged by a series of anxiety attacks, and tried to keep myself busy doing things so I wouldn't freak out. I felt like weeping on and off all day. Then, on day fourteen, I woke up super energized, went to the gym and my workout seemed effortless. I really felt like Harvoni was working and these lousy side effects I had the previous days seemed to be proof of the battle being won. Feeling good, I went online to see if the variety of highs and lows I had been experiencing was common among others.

"I have avoided treatment for 25 years, knowing the Hep C was eating away at my liver, but that the treatments were at best 50/50 and made you sick for 9 months. Then my doc was able to get me on the Harvoni program. I am over sixty, working a full week outdoors, and feel fine, no real side effects to report. I take the pill at night and wake up refreshed and ready to go at 5:30. I drink a lot of water and am watching what I eat. 59-year-old male."

"I'm a 44-year-old female. Started Harvoni ten days ago and had relatively no side effects except mild headaches. But

today, I have had pre-menopausal type heat flashes accompanied by trembling and fatigue, resulting in only 3-4 hours of sleep. I am cranky and emotional and have been crying off and on all day."

"I began the Harvoni treatment ten days ago and the worst part was the anxiety due to what I had experienced with interferon. Not much else to report."

"I have advanced fibrosis and am sixty years old. My biggest concern was how the Harvoni would affect my work and social life. But, if anything, I am more awake and able and have more energy. A couple tiny headaches here and there, but I drink water and they seem to go away. My future life looks promising!"

Gratitude for research scientists finally coming up with a low-impact cure for Hep C, was a theme reiterated time and again through all the message boards and chat rooms I visited. Hep C is such a debilitating disease that diminishes quality of life, it is easy to be grateful when a person can gain access to effective treatment with the promise of one day feeling normal.

"I have been hiding the fact that I have Hep C from everyone, even my closest friends. I'm on day 12 and it feels like I've had the flu for the past week, my muscles and joints ache, headache, nausea and insomnia. It's becoming harder for me to hide this from my family and close friends as they are starting to wonder what's wrong with me. Still, I am very

grateful that I was able to get on the program and that a cure is not too far away."

Several people complained about stomach acid problems and asked others what to do about it.

"I got Hep C from blood transfusions required during surgery in the 1980s. As tests for HCV were not perfected until 1992, there have been many lingering cases. Interferon didn't work and now Harvoni has the promise of being a miracle cure. I get acid reflux and had to stop taking Prilosec when I started Harvoni 11 days ago and have severe stomach acid pains. Anyone have any ideas what to do?"

I had asked my doctor and she told me not to take antacids, rather to dissolve a tablespoon of baking soda in an 8-ounce glass of water and drink it. It worked right way for me. However, two other people on the message boards offered positive suggestions from their own experiences and stated doctor recommendations. As always, check with your own doctor to be sure.

"My doctor said to wait at least 4 hours to take an antacid after taking Harvoni so the digestive system can better absorb the drug. Another thing that works is to take Harvoni before you go to sleep and take an antacid after your big meals, or eat smaller more frequent meals. You might look at what you are eating and see if changing your diet might cut down on the acid. You may have a food allergy."

"An alternative to Prilosec is Omeprazole. I take it when I take the Harvoni and haven't had any problems. But, check with your doctor, especially if you are taking any other medicine or supplements."

Drinking coffee during the Harvoni treatment was often a topic of discussion, as there are many reports available online about the beneficial properties of coffee on the human system including the liver. Whether these studies were funded by coffee growers or sellers is anyone's guess, so the best bet is always to ask your doctor. Here, people at various points in their treatment program, weighed in with their experiences about drinking coffee while taking Harvoni.

"I have read that the caffeine in coffee can exacerbate headaches you might get from Harvoni. However, my doctor told me to drink coffee for energy if the meds make me fatigued, so I guess it's all right."

"I have been drinking three cups in the morning every day since I started Harvoni and not noticed any effects from it."

"I noticed, from my own experience and from talking with others in the support room, that drinking coffee can either lessen or increase the severity of a headache. I think it depends on the individual person's severity of disease and physical health. I also have noticed that drinking plenty of water helps prevent headaches."

"I have been waiting 25 years for them to develop Harvoni and my viral loads were undetected after 4 weeks. My worst

side effect is fatigue and drinking coffee helps lift me out of the funk."

"I've been drinking four cups a day for years and didn't stop when I started Harvoni. No difference."

"Drinking lots of water is the answer to preventing Harvoni headaches from coffee or lessening the other common side effects."

Yes, drinking lots of water is one thing that every doctor and Harvoni user I have talked with, or seen comments from, have in common. You have to drink the recommended half gallon, gallon, or correct amount, of pure water every day to keep your body hydrated and help flush the dead Hep C cells from your system. The amount of water you need to optimally consume depends somewhat on your body weight, so take that into account. That a 95-pound female would need less water than a 250-pound man is just common sense. Looking over my collection of comments from the chat rooms, it is interesting to see how closely my experience parallels the experiences of others. For the remainder of this chapter I am going to show excerpts from my daily journal followed by comments from other people expressing what they are thinking and feeling at about the same point on the Harvoni journey.

Day 14… Feeling excellent. I went in and had my blood drawn for my two-week test. I also received a call from my doctor's office asking how I was feeling. That was really nice! I told them about the physical and psychological side effects I had been experiencing, and they said they were normal. I am beginning to feel comfortable with my daily routine and have adjusted to a certain amount of discomfort which can be lessened by drinking water, exercise and eating certain foods.

"Almost 2 weeks now. No real complaints. I have some days that I just am tired; occasional headache - but not enough that I require any over-the-counter meds. Lots of water really seems to help! If I feel a headache, I drink water. Just now beginning to feel discomfort in my right elbow when I bend. Very well pleased with the Drug. Diabetes is okay; I must monitor blood sugar levels extremely close."

"When I drink extra water I feel better. I learned that after the first week. I am crying more than normal, but am getting my period and that may have something to do with it. Also cut out soda. Yuk!"

Day 15... Feeling like my energy is increasing daily. It's so exciting to have energy like this when I have been feeling so shitty for years. Before Harvoni it was hard for me to move around for more than 20 minutes at a time before I had to go lay down. It was depressing. I felt my life was going to be limited into just staying around the house. It was like a box closing in on me, making my living space smaller and smaller. Now the box seems to be opening up, or like I am coming out of a long tunnel, the light at the end getting brighter and brighter.

"My headaches started out so bad they made me tired and I would fall asleep during the day. I also had the flu, but maybe flulike symptoms are a side effect of Harvoni. I also have had a dramatic increase in flatulence as after two weeks maybe my digestive system is ramping up with better functioning of my liver."

"I sometimes get dizzy spells after taking Harvoni and get headaches and hour after taking the tablet. Maybe I need to drink more water? I also am depressed and forgetful and can't remember if I had done a thing I started out to do. I get strange dreams too sometimes and don't want to get out of bed. I also am eating more and have increased a couple sizes in my jeans. Still, I am grateful of the cure and can't wait for it to be over."

"I'm eighty years old and have adjusted pretty well to the side effects of Harvoni. I get tired and have to plan activities around my naps. Loose bowels sometimes. No big deal." [80-years-old!]

Day 16… I have started noticing that I have no sex drive whatsoever, and today I feel bloated and a little depressed. I guess most people would feel this way if they didn't have a sexual release of any kind. This topic occasionally appears in Hep C support groups, and seems to concern some women more than others.

"A busy mother (44) under treatment, I am not feeling aroused at all. I wonder if my libido will come back after treatment."

"I'm 64 and sex right now is not a priority. Getting cured of Hep C is, so maybe I can live longer. I'll worry about sex later."

"I think worrying can diminish libido as much as anything. I have felt an increase in sexual drive, but it is not due to the Harvoni, rather my husband and I are spending more time together."

"I am more concerned about pleasing my husband than my own needs right now."

It was interesting how the women seemed more concerned about their partners, and how some men addressed the subject, often with a touch of humor or even an outright lie <g>.

"I'm in my ninth week and my sex drive has not improved any with the Harvoni. This is a bigger issue for me than my wife, but I want to keep her happy. I called my doctor's office and was told that Viagra was not on the list of meds that could interfere with Harvoni."

"Be careful about getting hormone replacement therapy for Low-T. I looked into it and decided to wait until I was off Harvoni for a couple months."

"We have been having sex three or four times a day. I hope when I get off Harvoni I can get back to the old routine of a couple times a week." [Yeah, right!]

"We're in our 60s and I felt a slight increase in libido once I got off Harvoni and was cured."

"I'm getting tired chasing my wife around the kitchen table. She is getting easier to catch though, she has a bad ankle."

"Worrying is enough to lower libido. ...My libido has gone down, but it's not the Harvoni."

"Three months post treatment and everything is back to normal."

"I am a few months post treatment I have experienced a sever loss of libido and the ability to maintain erections."

Consulting the Hepatitis Central website, I found several articles on libido and Hep C written by Nicole Cutler which nicely summarize current attitudes and findings.[2,3]

"Of the millions of people infected with HCV, many have a decreased interest in sex. Four of the most likely reasons for this association include:

<u>Depression</u> – Known to impair sex drive, clinical studies show that depression is significantly higher among HCV-infected patients compared with the general population.

<u>Fatigue</u> – Individuals with pronounced fatigue have little to no energy for sex. Chronic fatigue, the most commonly reported symptom of Hepatitis C infection, affects between 65 and 75 percent of those diagnosed with the disease.

Hormones – Most forms of chronic liver disease (including Hepatitis C) can alter hormone levels, providing a chemical basis for loss of libido.

Medications – The medications used to treat Hepatitis C are known to cause decreased libido; however, sex drive typically returns upon treatment cessation.[3]

Reading my fellow journeyers' comments and the general knowledge available on line, made me understand something very real: it was like a light bulb flashing on in my head. Harvoni is a very new drug, new enough to be considered somewhat in the experimental stage. The experiences we are sharing can be invaluable to doctors and researchers, as well as providing comfort and confidence to each other. We are on the front lines and will be for some time to come. Does it do any good to call our doctors with every little headache, itch, pain or worry? Seriously, doctors don't know all about Harvoni yet. For some of us, we are our doctor's first Harvoni patient. I am hoping the data we have collected and are sharing in this book, may be of service not only to my fellow dragon slayers on the Harvoni treatment trail, but also to researchers who may get an idea that will stimulate the formation of newer and better treatments. Time will tell.

Day 17… Feeling good, no changes. I was reading about people asking in the chat room if they have had any issues with their kidneys during Harvoni, if elevated sugar levels mean anything. In another support group someone said their doctor suggested only 20 grams of sugar a day as this somehow affected the electrolyte balance. Then I read that we should eat a lot of vegetables to keep our electrolytes in check. I wondered what electrolytes were and what they do, did some research on line and found that:

"An electrolyte is a substance that produces an electrically conducting solution when dissolved in water. Electrolytes carry a charge and are essential for life. Electrolytes regulate our nerve and muscle function, our body's hydration, blood pH, blood pressure, and the rebuilding of damaged tissue. Various mechanisms exist in our body that keep the concentrations of electrolytes under strict control. All higher forms of life need electrolytes to survive. In our bodies, electrolytes include sodium (Na+), potassium (K+), calcium (Ca2+), bicarbonate (HCO3-), magnesium (Mg2+), chloride (Cl-), and hydrogen phosphate (HPO42-). The level of an electrolyte in the blood can become too high or too low. Body electrolyte levels tend to alter when water levels in the body change - when our level of hydration goes up or down. Electrolyte levels are kept constant by our kidneys and several hormones. When we exercise we sweat and lose electrolytes, mainly sodium and potassium."[4]

This article also stated that fruits and vegetables are good sources of electrolytes, and that kidney disease and severe dehydration can cause electrolyte imbalance. This can result in a variety of symptoms, such as: irregular heartbeat, weakness, twitching, confusion, numbness, fatigue, moodiness and irritability, nausea lethargy, loss of appetite, constipation and muscle spasms. Ironically, I had experienced many of these symptoms during my course of Harvoni, as did many others in the online support groups. This made me realize how important eating fruits and vegetables, and drinking plenty of pure water, was in maintaining electrolyte balance, which in turn lessened the symptoms and facilitated the Hep C healing process. I credit following this strategy with the relatively mild side effects I had been experiencing, and what others were expressing in the support groups.

"I started Harvoni two weeks ago and have been having horrible headaches and debilitating fatigue. I have discovered a direct relationship between the level of pain and discomfort with what I eat and how much water I drink. It seems the key is to make digestion as easy as possible on the liver where the battle is raging. So I eat more fruits and vegetables – grapefruit, berries, apples, carrots, beets, avocados – and the side effects go way down. I also exercise and that helps a lot too."

Drinking lots of water is good, but not enough. You have to get your vitamins and minerals to keep those electrolytes in balance by eating plenty of fruits and vegetables, as my doctor said it was not wise to take any kind of vitamin or nutritional supplement while taking Harvoni.

Day 18… Woke up early as usual and took my Harvoni as soon as my eyes open with water which is abundant by my bedside. Then, a couple of hours later I am zipped like I am on speed or lots of caffeine. I know my liver is getting better, but am wondering if I will have days with killer energy (no pun intended) after I finish my round of treatment? Now it seems that lethargy becomes more sporadic than the norm. I really love it. I wonder if my good result is partially caused by other variables, like my good diet, exercise and water.

"I experienced no side effects the first week, but during the second and third weeks I got headaches, became fatigues and had occasional diarrhea. I drink 4 bottles (16.9 fl oz) a day, but I still feel thirsty. My body feels hot even in cold air-conditioning, I am irritable and emotionally fragile. Sometimes my eyes burn. I know I should exercise more, but don't know if that will help."

Day 19… Feeling full of energy, irritable and anxiety today, jittery.

Day 20… Feeling agitated again today, I can't put my finger on why I am feeling this way but have been noticing it a lot lately. I am usually pretty calm but for some reason there feels like an undercurrent going on deep inside, also feeling depressed, which I have noticed lessening during treatment but not altogether gone. There are just days when I feel like I am being pulled under water without air.

"My 20ᵗʰ day on Harvoni. No side effects until the 11ᵗʰ day. But, I have also had a cold. I don't know if the two are related, as maybe cold symptoms are similar to Harvoni symptoms. No fever, but fatigue, headaches and chills."

Day 21… Just when I thought I was out of the woods and everything was rosy, I get a slate of negative symptoms. I'm am wondering if they are physical or psychological or both. I went to the support groups and found solace in others expressing similar feelings about this same point in treatment.

"I have been very emotional about things the past two weeks on Harvoni. I've had acne and I seem to cry all the time for no reason."

"My Doctor prescribed Xanax to take only when needed for emotional stress, but I don't use it daily. Ask you doc if you are having anxiety attacks or other emotional issues."

Day 22… Sometimes the more research I do the more anxiety ridden I become. Do I have cirrhosis or not? Am I being healed to the extent of having no liver damage? Is my Hep C being cured so as not to prevent more liver scarring? Will the Hep C come back after I finish the 12 weeks of treatment? It's so scary and confusing sometimes not knowing about the true damage of my liver. Are other people besieged by worries today?

"I took interferon years ago, was cleared then the Hep C came back. I am now in my fourth week of Harvoni and the side effects are very minor. A headache one day, loose stool, but my eyes have cleared up and no fatigue. It may be because I go to the gym, work out for two hours, then drink a lot of water, come home and sleep. Coffee helps keep me alert during the day. My main concern is, if I get cleared will the Hep C come back?"

Day 23… I have been feeling really bloated and it seems that I haven't been able to eat much without feeling super full. So I have decided to just juice and drink Soylent as my main meals to see if my bloating will go down. Maybe I need to exercise more? I will try to go to the gym today.

Day 24… Today my stomach feels like I have hit every bar in town and drank each one of them dry. *The dragon is in me!* I have this horrible burning sensation. I took a little baking soda as I read that you shouldn't take Zantac or antacids. The burning feeling slowly died down, which made me feel like I was being reminded that the dragon being slayed had relatives hiding in other parts of my body where they are being routed from their nests.

"On my 23rd day. I had a headache the first day and a stomach ache the 2nd day and noticed a slight increase in blood pressure initially, but that could have been due to anxiety. I got HCV back in the 1970s, but was not diagnosed until 1992. I have had two liver transplants and hope the Harvoni can settle this thing once and for all."

"I am near my first month of Harvoni and have had some muscle soreness in my back and shoulders. I haven't seen much information on over-the-counter pain medicine. Anyone know anything about that?"

Day 25… The above question made me think about what my doctor had told me about over-the-counter pain killers. She told me Tylenol (acetaminophen) was okay despite its known effects on the liver, but to stay away from aspirin, Advil, Aleve and the others as they affected the kidneys more than the liver.[5] During Harvoni treatment, the kidneys needed to be kept in optimal shape to help remove the dead Hep C cells and other toxins. To make certain, I went to Google using the search words 'Harvoni + pain medicine' and found several articles of interest, a good one written by a registered nurse who stated:

"Once you've been diagnosed with a liver disease such as hepatitis C, many doctors will tell you not to take acetaminophen. However, talk to a hepatologist (a liver specialist), and they will tell you the opposite. When the liver is malfunctioning, it is unable to make clotting factors. NSAIDs increase bleeding risk. Also, cirrhosis is often accompanied by kidney failure, and NSAIDs are a no-no with poor functioning kidneys. Acetaminophen is used in liver transplant centers. Again, the key is to use it as directed."[6]

It's always best to go with the specialists. My doctor was absolutely correct. Even better than Tylenol were safer alternative ways to reduce headaches and other pain, as iterated by another author known for her numerous articles on many aspects of Hep C and treatment. These included: heat packs over muscles, joints or the liver; soak in a warm bath with Epsom salts; rub on a topical pain gel; get adequate rest as fatigue worsens pain; stretching or gentle exercise for muscle pain; go to a massage therapist, chiropractor or other qualified alternative professional.[5]

Day 26… I woke up feeling great, but as the morning went by I felt myself slide into an undeniable funk. I have some really sad family issues going on and it is immobilizing me for sure. All that crosses my mind is that the Hep C will return and this adding to my depression. It will pass I know it will. I find meditation to be one of the most helpful tools that I know, it helps one cope when stress levels hit the roof. Twenty minutes in the morning and 20 in the afternoon, I try my best to be diligent making it part of my daily routine... I try.

Day 27... I woke up hungry today and had a big bowl of granola cereal which gave me energy and made me feel better. Maybe I shouldn't be taking the Harvoni on an empty stomach first thing in the morning, but I heard it works better when it is in your stomach alone. Anyway, that has been my method and I'm sticking to it.

"I'm on my 4th week of Harvoni. I was very hungry during the third week and ate like crazy, then the urge stopped. Then I began to feel bloated coupled with constipation and have a hard time sleep. My body is definitely going through changes. It feels like my liver has begun functioning normally again."

Day 28... End of the fourth week. Today I go in for my next blood test. I am anxious to see my results. I expect to be undetected as I am doing everything by the book. The thought of this makes me feel better. Just eight more weeks to go!

WEEKS 5-12:
Good Days and Bad Days

The second of three bottles of Harvoni was delivered overnight to my door by FedEx before 10:30 a.m. on the day before the first bottle would be empty. The cheerful disposition of the driver who asked me to sign, seemed a good omen that everything was progressing right on schedule and I was on my way to being cured. I zipped open the big envelope with the bright orange and purple lettering and pulled out the bottle. It was still amazing to me that I held such a valuable cache of pharmaceuticals in my hand.

The second and third month of taking Harvoni was basically a repeat of the first month, except that I had become adjusted to the daily routine that had characterized my life. Also, my viral load had been reduced to undetectable, so I was feeling better due to the decreased harmful effects caused by HCV. This was a similar experience for many of my online friends. But, even though we felt better, it was important to continue on Harvoni for the next eight weeks and complete the treatment. My doctor compared this to finishing the full prescribed dosage of antibiotics when a person was fighting pneumonia or some other infection.

"I have been on Harvoni for 5 weeks and feel like I am on an emotional roller coaster. I have the typical side effects of a slight headache and constipation, tiredness and a slight headache once in great while. I go to bed early after taking

Harvoni at 6 p.m., sleep like a baby and wake up early. Though my viral counts are undetected, I need seven more weeks of the same routine to effect the cure."

Those who had previously done an early Hep C treatment with interferon / ribavirin seemed to have a harder time than those of us who were treatment-naïve.

"I have gone through treatment twice that didn't work, first with interferon and ribavirin, then with interferon, ribavirin and Incivek. I'm on my second month of Harvoni and have had typical side effects of fatigue, nausea, depression, but they eased up after the third week. I have been trying to cure this disease since 1975 and hope the Harvoni will work. Never again will I take those other toxic poisons."

Many people felt as I did and were able to continue on with their normal lives, experiencing very few side effects, or coping with them as need be. Others were not as lucky due to genetics, or not being as conscientious in such things as drinking lots of water, eating right, or exercising.

"I have gained weight and feel lousy most of the time. I have headaches and take ibuprofen almost every day. I often cry for no reason, get stomach cramps, diarrhea and nausea. I started grinding my teeth at night and never did that before. It's discouraging that I seem to be in the small percentage of Harvoni takers who get severe side effects. It's just my 5th week and I have 7 more to go!"

My third month was basically a repeat of the second month with up and down days, pain in different areas of my body. Sometimes I would concentrate on the pain coming from a joint or an organ and could visualize the Harvoni attacking the hiding virus like a squad of Lilliputian soldiers. But, I had read so much and was so into getting cured, I'm sure my imagination played a role. I had been through so much pain and suffering through the years, it seemed like the veil that had clouded my vitality was dissolving daily. I religiously took the tablet in the morning, had a simple breakfast of granola, my fresh juice concoction for lunch, and Soylent or a simple meal for dinner. And, of course, lots of pure water.

"Have had Hep C for 35 years and am in week 9 of 12. I take Harvoni at night, sleep well and wake up early. I realized drinking a gallon of water a day helps the Harvoni adsorb and helps decrease side effects. I got headaches first few days as I didn't drink water. My diet consist of vegetables, fish, whole grain, fruit and dark chocolate. If you manage your water, diet and exercise, the side effects are minimal."

Occasionally my mate and I went out for a meal, but he lives like a Spartan, surviving on a simple breakfast, exercise about 2 p.m. then his main meal, then maybe some fruit in the evening. He went on a simple diet with me and lost about 25 pounds in two months. He also remained free of alcohol to give me support and it really helped, though he is a bit of a stoic and doesn't complain. One time he had a fragmented disc in his lower back and suffered for two months before he sought surgical help, thinking he could repair it himself through yoga. He has always been there for me when I really needed him, but didn't cater much to complaints. This bolstered my courage to face up to whatever each day would bring and live through it. This also gave me perspective on how other people in the support groups viewed their Harvoni experiences, how much they took in stride and how much they were given to complain.

"I have diabetes, am 49-years-old, work full time at a gym, never had to take off a day of work and have had very few side effects after eight weeks. I did notice an appetite increase."

"16 days left in my 8-week treatment plan. My viral load was undetected after week three. I've had mild headaches, muscle aches, fatigue, and insomnia. Going to the gym helps remove the aches."

"I have irritable bowel syndrome (IBS) and ulcerative colitis that are currently in remission, and the Harvoni has not produced any change in the way I feel."

"I've been taking Harvoni for nine weeks and have had some side effects not many others seem to have, namely a rash on my face and hair loss. I am emotional and get upset for no apparent reason. Those of you who don't report any real problems are very lucky."

"My 8th week and the increased energy I have had has resulted in insomnia. People have told me insomnia is not a side effect, but I looked up the 31-page Harvoni info sheet

online and see insomnia is one of the five most common side effects."

Yes, as this person mentioned, there are five main side effects cited in the product literature that is readily available on the Harvoni website (see reference at end of book]. Main side effects from Harvoni are fatigue, headache, nausea, diarrhea and insomnia. The table below shows the typical side effects and percentage of treatment patients affected in 8, 12 and 24 week studies [N = number of participants].[1]

Harvoni Users Reported Major Adverse Reactions / Treatment Length			
	8 weeks N = 215	**12 weeks** N = 539	**24 weeks** N = 326
Fatigue	16%	13%	18%
Headache	11%	14%	17%
Nausea	6%	7%	9%
Diarrhea	4%	3%	7%
Insomnia	3%	5%	6%

Because of my genotype and diagnosis, my treatment length was 12 weeks, though my viral load and stats had basically returned to within normal ranges in the first month and remained there. Some patients with less severe cases were prescribed an eight-week treatment plan, which seemed to work just fine.

"My eight weeks are done and the side effects are disappearing, though the extra energy has caused sleeplessness. But, normal sleep is retuning. I am very grateful for a cure that is not chemotherapy."

"I just finished eight weeks of treatment, but was clear after three weeks. My doctor said I can't be considered 'cured' until the bloodwork three months after the treatment ends shows clear."

While the usual length of treatment is eight or twelve weeks, some cases required 24 weeks. This seemed to be mostly true for those who were treatment-experienced, or whose liver disease was more advanced.

"With interferon / ribavirin I was plagued by serious anemia, weakness, fatigue and depression, exacerbated from knowing the treatment was failing and I had to go to work no matter how horrible I felt. This 24 weeks on Harvoni has been a breeze and it works! My loads are undetectable at 12 weeks, but I will continue to finish the treatment to the end to make sure."

Some of my fellow dragon slayers did not have the same responses treatment as the majority of us, and the HCV remained potent in their blood streams. This caused their physicians to modify the prescribed treatment regimen by either extending the length of treatment or adding a secondary drug.

"My viral load was still detectable at 5 weeks, so my doctor added another 12 weeks, making my total treatment to be 24 weeks."

"I've been on Harvoni for 12 weeks with minimal sides, but am still detectable, so my doc has added ribavirin to my Harvoni for another 12 weeks. I did interferon years ago for an entire year and was beat down to the ground. This Harvoni is a cake walk."

"My treatment plan called for 12 weeks of Harvoni. He added ribavirin at 12 weeks as a viral load was still detected."

In one case, the person's system was so sensitive, and the side effects so pronounced, the Harvoni dosage had to be cut in half and the treatment period extended.

"I was having major side effects, massive headaches, extreme fatigue and severe brain fog, so my doctor cut my dose in half and doubled the length of treatment form 8 weeks to 16 weeks. I only weigh 135 pounds, so that may have something to do with it. I learned that staying properly hydrated helps a lot."

Day 84, August 1, 2016… I awakened at 6:36 and took my last pill. I could not believe how fast the 12 weeks flew by. I was simultaneously relieved and apprehensive. What now? What if my new found energy diminishes? What if I get a whole new set of side effects? What if the Hep C comes back?

Uncertainty breeds fear and these thoughts were born from not really knowing what to expect. Sure, I had read all about it and spent countless hours in the online support groups, but now I was out of the woods with a clear road ahead of me and didn't know which way to go. My mate/mentor/coach reiterated the old adage "idle hands are the devil's workshop," and I knew keeping busy was the best way to forget about my worries and slide gracefully into my new state of being HCV free. All in all, I felt grateful that I was able to take advantage of the treatment and that the one pill a day Harvoni was so more effective than the interferon treatment many people suffered through just a few years ago with a 50% chance of cure.

"I took the interferon / ribavirin treatment 16 years ago and it was brutal. I lost most of my hair, 25 pounds, couldn't sleep and it didn't work. On the contrary, Harvoni is great. I've finished treatment and virus free. If you are starting Harvoni, have faith in the fact that it works!"

The day after my last pill I was scheduled to get my blood drawn at the lab to check my viral load, then again a month later. I grew apprehensive that my doctor would discover something in the results that would indicate I was in the small percentage of people who didn't get cured and I would have to go back into treatment. What will she tell me? I know she can't really say I am "cured" until six months after completion of treatment. This is a bitter sweet milestone for me. I feel like I have done everything I'm supposed to do for the Harvoni to have worked its magic, tons of water, exercise, rest, juicing, hardly any red meat, mostly fish or chicken. I've noticed in the chat rooms people who have become undetected within the first month are as elated as people who state that they are cured 6 months post treatment. My worries vanished when my doctor said my stats were good and the HCV was undetected.

My diagnosis was HCV genotype 1a, treatment-naïve without cirrhosis. I was lucky that my Harvoni treatment only lasted twelve weeks, my viral loads were undetectable and other significant blood criteria were back within normal ranges. After twelve weeks I, with many others, moved into the post-treatment phase where the Harvoni began to leave our systems and we would rapidly stabilize our body chemistry without the deleterious effects of the Hep C virus.

However, some of the others who were treatment-experienced, who had cirrhosis or other more severe HCV criteria mentioned earlier, were prescribed 24-week treatment programs. To read about their perceptions about this extended treatment, you might visit some of the chat rooms and message boards presented in the resources section at the end of this book.

POST TREATMENT – What Next?

It was a bit of a shock to wake up on the 85th day and not have a Harvoni tablet sitting next to the bottle of water by my bedside. I got up in a kind of daze, studying the way I felt. I realized that Harvoni had been a kind of security blanket I had with me for 12 weeks, now it was gone and I had to live without it. It had done its job according to my blood test results, and I read it would still be in my system for a couple weeks, but had it really effected a permanent cure so my viral load levels would remain undetected? I hoped and prayed it would be so.

As I got ready for my first follow-up doctor appointment, I noticed my hair was thinner, and that my weight had dropped from 175 to 159 pounds. I attributed this to changing my diet to juicing and cutting out carbs like bread. This resulted in having more energy to go to the gym, which also helped. But, above all, I felt my liver had thrown off the shackles Hep C so it was working optimally. I noticed my food was digesting quicker with less stress and that my bloating went down as well as my flatulence.

My mouth felt dry and I drank a bottle of water, perhaps the bottle I had missed from not having to take the Harvoni. I missed the usual rush of energy the Harvoni gave me first thing in the morning and started to feel fatigued. I wondered if this was physical or psychological. I had the worry that without Harvoni my fatigue would return full blown but, as I started moving around, my energy seemed to come back. All in all it had been a very good ending thus far to 12 weeks of treatment.

I went to my doctor's office for the first follow-up appointment and she was very sweet and informative. My labs came back and my panel is still within the normal range. My next appointment is in 6 months where they will do a scan of my liver to determine if I have cirrhosis, my stage of fibrosis, and the probability of how much my liver will rejuvenate over time. She and I discussed how sad it is that Harvoni and the other effective drugs are not readily available to everyone in this country due to their high cost, but we were hopeful as time passed agreements could be made between the drug manufactures, the insurance companies, and the governmental health agencies to make it possible to eradicate this epidemic. She said a movement is underway to help bring these changes into effect.

After I got home I visited an online Harvoni support group to see if anyone else had just ended their treatment cycle and how they felt.

"No detectable Hep C after 12 weeks and my viral loads went from 21,000,000 down to zero! I gained 8 pounds and mild insomnia. I experimented and found after dinner is the best time to take the Harvoni pill. Drinking a gallon of water every day kept the headaches to a minimum and lessened the fatigue. I tried interferon once before, the side effects were horrible and it didn't work. Putting on a few pounds and losing a sleep was worth it to be rid of Hep C!"

The second day post-treatment I awoke still expecting to take the Harvoni pill. It has been my discipline for 12 weeks and now things have moved on to the next phase. It's an odd feeling as I would be so full of anticipation that the end was drawing near and I was becoming healthier and healthier. I was spending more time monitoring what others were saying about post Harvoni side effects, and found that many others were having the similar experiences.

"My first couple of weeks after Harvoni treatment I felt very tired, had a sore throat, and muscle aches like I had the flu. I got a lot of sleep and rest and my symptoms disappeared and my energy came back. Now I feel great!"

"It seemed there were some withdrawal symptoms from Harvoni, including tiredness, constipation, mood swings. But these faded away and I felt better after a couple weeks."

"The side affects others mention while taking Harvoni, I got after I finished twelve weeks of treatment and my viral load was undetectable – headaches, fatigue – but I think it was just my body readjusting. I continued drinking a gallon of water a day and that helped. Much much easier than interferon that didn't work. Gained a few pounds, but they came off pretty quick."

I kept thinking positive that I would not have the after effects some had expressed, but I did feel super fatigued. I was supposed to volunteer at the hospital, but could not muster the energy to get dressed, nor was my mood in any condition to deal with anything or anyone. My agitation and anxiety about minor things was going through the roof. So, I dropped everything and took my dog for a long walk in the park, hoping it would let things pass. I tried to make myself feel grateful I had waited for Harvoni to come on the market and did not seek treatment back in the days when interferon was the only option. I drank a lot of water and had a nap.

The third day Harvoni post treatment, I woke up in a great mood and felt very rested. I regarded the previous days' panic attacks as being my 'water under the bridge,' and was glad I took the long walk and detached from any responsibilities I was not ready to handle. Battling Hep C with Harvoni was a major life event, accompanied by all sorts of physical, psychological and emotion issues. All those years I suffered with worsening symptoms of the disease and, now to have them obliterated, was a lot to comprehend in a short time. I read it takes about 10-14 days for the Harvoni to leave your system fully after treatment and there is doubtlessly a range of side effects to be expected and recognized for what they are. I simply had to deal with them.

"The Harvoni literature says it takes about 12 days for the Harvoni to be cleansed out of the blood stream. I am 14 days post treatment, have no more headaches, my eyes are clear and my digestive system seems to be working better than I can remember. I feel good!"

That evening we went to dinner at a good friend's home I had a couple of glasses of wine just to check and see what would happen. In the past with Hep C full blown in my system, I would wake up the next day with blood shot eyes, have a burning sensation in my stomach area and feel very sluggish and mentally foggy. The next morning I woke up with white eyes, full of good energy and no feeling whatsoever in my stomach area. My liver was back functioning as normal as could be expected. This confirmed the fact that I am undetected, and when I receive a full clean bill of health I can enjoy a social drink occasionally. I do enjoy my wine with friends and dinner and my doctor said it would be okay to have a couple glasses every once in a while, but not to overdo it. I had faithfully abstained during the 12 weeks of Harvoni treatment and the results were worth it.

"I started treatment anticipating it would take 12 weeks, but since I had never had treatment before after my blood results came back my doctor cut it to eight weeks. I had Hep C since for 25 years and never let it stop me from enjoying a little wine or beer. I never did any drugs. But, during the treatment period I abstained. My side effects were few, a couple night sweats and slight headaches. I had a tooth extraction and that was worse than the Harvoni."

On the fifth day post treatment, I received a letter in the mail reminding me to get more labs done on the 30th of August. I am so pleased and grateful for the care I received from my doctor, and how I have been treated by my health care team throughout this process. They have done miracles in helping me overcome the psychological stigma attached to Hep C, regarding it strictly as a medical and scientific problem and leaving any discoloration from moral or social misinformation out of it.

Today I was able to play eighteen holes of golf with a girlfriend and found it effortless, even though the weather started to bake around the 15th hole. I came home energized and happy. I feel so blessed that my body was functioning so well, something I I have missed for so many years. When I would play pre-treatment, exhaustion would hit me like a ton of bricks when I walked 9 holes, never mind riding 18. It felt so good to be BACK!!!!

In fact, everything I did no matter what it was, cleaning, running errands, or just playing with my granddaughter, I always needed rest in between every single activity. My poor grandchild would have to be happy just lying on the bed with me reading or drawing or otherwise occupying herself. She is so sweet to have fully understood I just couldn't keep up with her due to my ill health. I no longer have to monitor my activities, I just do them without worrying.

It did take some getting used to, from having no energy to having energy. I sometimes felt like pinching myself I felt so good. Because my system was so clean from healing, juicing and exercising, I had to start drinking decaf because a cup of coffee would send me through the roof with boundless energy. Now, I just use coffee for a pick me up and drink decaf for the flavor. During the Harvoni treatment on this diet I lost 16 pounds.

"I have been clear for 9 months and am still working on losing the 20 pounds I gained during treatment. It took a few weeks until I had the energy to exercise and now walk almost every day. Don't worry about the weight until your treatment is complete, then you can work off the pounds."

I remember finding comfort in the comment above and thought when my treatment was over I would take a similar approach and lose the weight. Unfortunately, there are some people who had problems outside the usual range of those reported.

"I had to take Harvoni for 24 weeks. I gained 20 pounds of bulging lumpy fat starting about week 6. I finished Harvoni a couple months ago and am still gaining weight. Nothing I do seems to stop it. I've been walking, doing yoga, stretching, swimming, and have been on the Mediterranean diet for 15 years. I also feel worse now in the joints, have more irritability and brain fog than I did before I took the first pill. Very regretful I took the drug."

"You are not alone. I experienced the same side effects as you. But now I'm negative for Hep C. It's worth it!!"

Sixth day post-treatment I was in such a funk I couldn't function very well. I went out and ran errands. I don't think it was the let down from the intense psychological focus I had enjoyed with the Harvoni, but with other personal issues related to my children. I realize that for the past several years when the Hep C was the worse, I have been erratic and inconsistent with my daughters in many ways. This has led to confusion and many misunderstandings that will take some time to rectify. I realize this has also been a strain for my mate and my up-and-down personality has caused him to develop a kind of insensitive and calloused attitude regarding my extreme mood swings. He told me one time, "No one knows what you are going to do next." Well, it was true. I just have to own up to it and, hopefully, over the not too distance future, my stabilized behavior will come to be accepted as the new norm and things will work themselves out. But, after having gone through this experience and sharing it with others, I realize my behavior was not uncommon among people with HCV gnawing away at their insides.

"I never associated my depression, fatigue, and exhaustion with Hep C, because I didn't know any better. I just thought it was a natural part of my lunacy. After joining this group, only then did it start making sense that what I was feeling was "normal" among Hep C sufferers."

Sunday, 7th day post-treatment… I woke up feeling better, thank goodness. I wrote in my journal for a couple hours with coffee, then had a shower and took my dog for a nice long walk around the Arboretum. That made me feel a whole lot better. Getting up and doing things makes me feel better. It's kind of strange having the energy and not feeling sick all the time. It was like I was conditioned not to be able to do things. I realized now I had to change my entire orientation, that I could expand my range of activities, that I could make commitments to do things I could keep. It was a wonderful, yet scary revelation. It was like my world that had been closed off for so long was finally opened to me again. The way I felt was summarized nicely by one of my fellow dragon slayers.

"I thought through the years I had done a lot of damage to myself and my life would be short. I also broke into tears when my doctor told me I was cured. I am so grateful to

Harvoni and all the people who supported me online in this group. You helped me face my fears and worries and forge me into a dragon slayer! Now, I want to help others do the same. Thank you, thank you."

Day 8 post TX… Woke up feeling great. My daughter has to go for a training on the west coast so I have my five-year-old precocious granddaughter for five days straight. This will be a test of my endurance. In the past, after I had her for a day or two, I would have to recuperate the next day by mostly sleeping. So, I am excited to see how it goes this week. My expectations are not going to be too high because I am 61. Ask any grandmother my age and they will tell you the reason we have children when we are younger is because we have more energy for them. So I know it's going to be exhausting but hopefully not debilitating within the first few hours. She loves to visit as we play all day, go shopping, draw, read books – she is a ball of positive energy and a real joy. I took some vitamins to see if they might help, as I read they did help others post-treatment.

"After treatment I began experiencing weakness and shortness of breath and took myself to urgent care. They didn't find anything wrong, but suggested I start taking some vitamin D3. I bought some and began feeling better in a couple days. This leads me to think that once the liver starts functioning like it should demands for nutrients and food breakdown catalysts become higher. I recommend everyone investigate the right type and amount of supplements for themselves."

Day nine and I was feeling fine! I went out with my granddaughter yesterday, didn't have to take a break in playtime or shopping time, but when it turned 7:30 I was like ready for the 8 o'clock bedtime to roll around. It was the first night before the start of the new school year. We laid her clothes out on the ironing board and got her backpack ready by the door. She was going into the first grade at the same school where she attended kindergarten the year before and had a wonderful experience. We had such a great time the day before, and I held up so well, I felt could do the same. But, after I drop her at school I had the day to myself and wanted to go into the Harvoni support rooms and see how the others we coping post-treatment.

I found a section of postings in a new room I hadn't seen before about possible side effects I think it is important to mention, even though they affect only a small percentage of those who go on the Harvoni regimen. One concern was kidney disease and, although it was not directly related to Harvoni, it was linked to having HCV. The longer the Hep C virus remains active in your system, the greater the likelihood disease can migrate to other organs, such as the kidneys. I researched this subject online and found the following scientific report:

"Over time, untreated infections can lead to kidney disease: hepatitis C is no exception. Given the circumstances of HCV, it's possible that the virus may affect other organs, like the kidneys, without your knowledge. Early detection of hepatitis C may decrease the risk of the infection spreading to other organs in the body. Symptoms include: loss of appetite, dark

urine, diarrhea, nausea, stomach pain, excessive fatigue, jaundice (a yellowing of the skin and eyes)."[1]

I made a mental note to be on alert for these symptoms and to ask my doctor about kidney disease, and what blood tests might be an indication that something could be going wrong. Another concern of some of my fellow journeyers involved the heart.

"I have been experiencing shortness of breath, chest pains and what seems to be an irregular heartbeat. I have been finished with Harvoni for 12 weeks and having anxiety that may be causing my blood pressure to spike. I am seeing a hypertension doctor am on blood pressure medication. I don't know if there is a correlation between Harvoni and the heart, but need to find out."

Anything to do with the heart is a serious concern, and both Gilead and the FDA have issued strong statements about using Harvoni in combination with drugs prescribed to treat ventricular arrhythmias (abnormal heart rhythm). Serious problems have occurred, even death, when Harvoni has been used with Amiodarone.[2,3,4,5,6] This warning is clearly stated in the Harvoni insert literature:

"Bradycardia with amiodarone coadministration: Serious symptomatic bradycardia may occur in patients taking amiodarone, particularly in patients also receiving beta blockers, or those with underlying cardiac comorbidities and/or advanced liver disease. Coadministration of amiodarone with HARVONI is not recommended. In patients

without alternative, viable treatment options, cardiac monitoring is recommended."[7]

It should be noted that smoking cigarettes while taking Harvoni might be the cause of spiked heart rhythm. Or, it could even be caused by the simple anxiety caused by all the psychological considerations about treatment. Regardless, any noticeable change in heartbeat rate, pulse strength, or other indicators should be mentioned immediately to your doctor.

"I am overweight, smoke about half a pack a day and think my heart palpitations may be as caused by the nicotine as anything else."

Day 11… I felt nauseated most of the day with headaches, I attribute this to no caffeine, because I was drinking too much coffee and was flying off the walls with my heightened sensitivity. So when I decided to taper back and drink decaf, I felt like crap. Also my craving for bread came back which has made me feel sluggish. And, being on the fifth day with my granddaughter is taking its toll. I am not as young as I used to be! But, I am grateful Harvoni gave me back my energy and I had a wonderful time. Being with her reinforced the notion that being a mother was the highlight of my life. I loved being a mom and realize now that I have had a void in my life since my daughters grew up, left home and divorced themselves from us.

Day 12… this is the day they say Harvoni should be out of my system, and I am feeling a little tired. Maybe it's from the whole ordeal of thinking about the cure, thinking about being able to get the cure, getting approved for the cure, the twelve weeks of going through treatment with all its ups and downs, and now, that's it all over, I have a void there, similar to what I feel about my children. I need to find something meaningful to do with all this new found energy. It is such a recent phenomenon in my life, it is going to take some getting used to.

Looking back over my Harvoni experience, I can say it has been a real trip with amazing results. I had some good days, some bad days, but mostly just normal on-the-road-to-be-cured days. I think my liver is functionally normally and I can tell by the way my food digests, how clear my eyes are and how my energy level has gone way up. I didn't realize how hampered I had been all these years. I will be grateful for this cure for the rest of my life (which has been extended by many years, I hope!).

AFTERWARD – Am I Really Cured?

One thing my doctor, and many others I have spoken with, caution me about is thinking that I am "cured" of the Hepatitis C virus. Though my AST, ALT, and APT numbers may be back in range and my HCV/RNA may be undetected, I must never think that I am totally cured of the disease. As long as I live there will always be a minute trace of the dragon inside my body which will, hopefully, lay dormant and never again raise its ugly head. I had not thought about the distinction between being 'cleared' of the virus and being 'cured.' Here is an explanation from one of my fellow dragon slayers I found to be particularly relevant which seems to reflect the current science:

Clearing the Virus vs Being Cured

Clearing the virus or when the virus is undetected, means that the virus is not detected in a small sample of the blood. SVR (sustained viral load) or cure means the virus remains undetected, 3 to 6 months post treatment. This is a very important distinction because the virus is very strong and extremely SNEAKY. This is why it has taken so long to develop a drug that works so well. It is very important to continue to take the meds even if the virus is no longer detected after a short time on treatment. It is not unlike your doctor telling you to continue taking a round of antibiotics even if you are feeling better in a few days. You need to finish your meds. The virus is measured in hundredths of thousands or millions per tiny amount of blood that is drawn. This is where the viral load comes from. That's the amount of virus in that tiny portion.

The virus can hide out anywhere in your body, not just in your liver or your blood. It can hide in your spleen and soft tissue as well, this is why we continue to test 3 - 6 months post treatment, to make absolutely sure it is gone. We need to drink plenty of water not only to stay hydrated, but to flush the dead virus and toxins from our bodies.

There will be a certain number of people that relapse. The cure rates are 93-98%, depending on your diagnosis. We need to remain positive because most of us will reach SVR (sustained viral response). We will be free of this disease and get our lives back.

A cure, in medical terms, is defined as a sustained virologic response (SVR) determined when no HCV/RNA is detected in the blood 24 weeks after treatment is completed. Data has shown in long term follow-up studies that persons who achieve SVR after six months are considered to be "cured" virologically.[1,2] But, not everyone gets cured on the first treatment and may have to do it again with a different combination of drugs. Even if you do not become "cured" after the first treatment, there are still real benefits to be enjoyed.

"While the goal of HCV therapy is to effectively eradicate the virus and to live a healthy, hepatitis-free life, you shouldn't despair if you are unable to achieve these goals. Even if you only have partial response, studies have shown that the benefits to the liver can be profound, not only slowing the course of the disease but in some cases reversing fibrosis even in those with marked liver damage."[1]

Term	Meaning	Definition	Prognosis
RVR	Rapid viral response	An undetectable viral load after four weeks of treatment	Generally more likely to achieve SVR
eRVR	Extended rapid viral response	An undetectable viral load at week 12, following the initial RVR	Generally more likely to achieve SVR
EVR	Early viral response	An undetectable viral load or a 99% reduction in viral load by week 12	More important as a predictor of treatment outcome as failure to achieve EVR correlates to less than 4% chance of achieving SVR
ETR	End of treatment response	An undetectable viral load achieved by the end of week 12	Not helpful in predicting treatment outcomes
Partial responder		Able to achieve EVR but unable to sustain an undetectable viral load 24 weeks after therapy completion	Considered treatment failure
Null responder		Unable to achieve EVR by week 12	Treatment is typically terminated if EVR is not achieved by week 12
SVR	Sustained viral response	Able to sustain undetectable viral load for 12 weeks (SVR-12) and 24 weeks (SVR-24) following completion of therapy	SVR-24 is considered a "cure," while patients with SVR-12 are usually able to achieve SVR-24

Charles Daniel provides an excellent summary of the medical terminology with definitions and prognosis as indicated in the table above.[1]

Research in Phase III human trials has shown that the different Hep C drugs on the market today have proven extremely effective, for both treatment-experienced and treatment-naïve patients, compared to the interferon / ribavirin treatment programs which were initially devised to fight the disease years ago:

Daklinza with **Sovaldi**: 98% naive and 58% experienced with cirrhosis.

Harvoni 99% naïve and 94% experienced.

Sovaldi with ribavirin + peginterferon or ribavirin alone: 82% to 92% overall.

Technivie: 99% naïve and experienced.

Viekira Pak: 95% naïve and experienced.

Olysio with ribavirin + peginterferon: 80% to 85% naïve.

Zepatier with or without ribavirin: 95% naïve and experienced.[1]

Once a person achieves SVR and is "cleared" of Hepatitis C, the odds of the virus returning are extremely small. Unlike viruses such as chicken pox, Hepatitis A or the measles, which produce antibodies and create immunity to future infection, antibodies formed to combat Hep C do not contain this characteristic. It is possible for you to acquire the Hep C virus again if you come into contact with an untreated infected person and have a blood-to-blood transfer. Thus, it is important that you do not engage in any of these high risk behaviors:

- Sharing needles used for intravenous drugs or tattoos.
- Snorting drugs with shared equipment.
- Sharing personal care items (toothbrush, razor, etc.) with an infected person.
- Engaging in high-risk sexual behavior with an infected partner.[2]

In short, the more time that passes after you have achieved SVR, the more confidence you can have in the idea that you are "cured." And, the way you feel will be an important indicator for the rest of your life. If you ever are in doubt, see your doctor.

I was also curious if there was any chance I might be able to infect others once I achieved SVR, and found this statement:

"In general, we are more comfortable living in a world of absolutes than acknowledging several shades of grey. Unfortunately, the potential for infectivity following a Hepatitis C cure lies somewhat in the grey category... experts' opinions on this matter vary." [3]

So, no one really knows for sure. The best course of action is to be careful. Be vigilant of your behavior and the behavior of others you associate with.

A final thought, and this is important. You have lived with the rigors of Hep C for years, some of you for decades. You know what having the HCV inside your body is like, how it robs your energy, precipitates mood swings, causes brain fog and the whole host of symptoms we have been discussing in this book. What if you had gotten tested when you first contracted the disease, entered treatment right away and gotten cured? How would your life have been different these past many years?

Of course, Harvoni and the other modern one-pill cures were not available years ago, but they are today. And, treatment can be over in as little as eight weeks by watching your diet, drinking plenty of water and taking one tablet a day. A major concern among many people I have spoken with in the online support groups, was stated succinctly by this person:

"For the first time since 1985, I'm not afraid that I may pass this disease on to someone I love. All those years I had Hep C multiplying in my system made me a walking hazard. Thank God that is over!"

This is why you should tell everyone you have been in contact with – friends, lovers, siblings, children – to go get tested for Hep C right away. The test is simple, inexpensive and thorough. You have taken responsibility for your own cure, now you can extend your gratitude by helping others. It is a real possibility that Hep C can be eradicated in a generation or two, just like polio. But, it will take a concerted effort of everyone working together.

In closing, we want to thank you for reading this book. We hope you feel more knowledgeable and better informed about Hep C, Harvoni and the other 'miracle' drugs now available. We have worked hard to make sure all the information in this book is correct and up-to-date. Please write to: comments@theharvoniexperience.com.

RESOURCES

If you want more detailed information on other aspects of Hepatitis C and treatment options, the following list of references may be helpful. While every effort has been made to verify the workability of these links, links do get broken and change over time, so we recommend you perform a current Google search for current information on any topic of interest.

Basic Information
- Hepatitis C (Mayo Foundation for Medical Education and Research)
- Hepatitis C (National Institute of Allergy and Infectious Diseases)
- Hepatitis C FAQs (Centers for Disease Control and Prevention)
- What I Need to Know about Hepatitis C (National Institute of Diabetes and Digestive and Kidney Diseases) Also in Spanish

News Articles
- Sharing Drug 'Snorting Straws' Spreads Hepatitis C (07/27/2016, HealthDay)
- Epclusa Approved for Chronic Hepatitis C (06/28/2016, HealthDay)
- Hepatitis C Patients More Likely to Drink, Study Finds (05/25/2016, HealthDay)

Diagnosis and Tests

- CDC Vital Signs: Hepatitis C: Testing Baby Boomers Saves Lives (Centers for Disease Control and Prevention)
- Hepatitis C Screening in the Behavioral Healthcare Setting (Substance Abuse and Mental Health Services Administration)
- Hepatitis C Test (American Association for Clinical Chemistry)
- Hepatitis C: What to Expect When Getting Tested (Centers for Disease Control and Prevention) - PDF
- Know More Hepatitis (Centers for Disease Control and Prevention)
- Liver Biopsy (National Institute of Diabetes and Digestive and Kidney Diseases) Also in Spanish
- Liver Panel (American Association for Clinical Chemistry)

Treatments and Therapies

- Alternative and Complementary Therapies for Hepatitis C (Department of Veterans Affairs)
- CAM and Hepatitis C: A Focus on Herbal Supplements (National Center for Complementary and Integrative Health)
- Hepatitis C: Treatment (Department of Veterans Affairs)
- Patient Treatment Tracking Chart (Department of Veterans Affairs)
- Time to Talk: 5 Things You Should Know about Dietary Supplements for Hepatitis C (National Center for Complementary and Integrative Health)

Living With Hep C

- Hepatitis C: Diet and Nutrition (Department of Veterans Affairs)
- Hepatitis C: Managing Pain (Department of Veterans Affairs)
- Hepatitis C: Mental Health (Department of Veterans Affairs)
- Tips to Lessen Common Side Effects of HCV Therapy (American College of Gastroenterology) - PDF

Related Issues

- Alcohol and Hepatitis C (Department of Veterans Affairs)
- HCV and Rheumatic Disease (American College of Rheumatology)
- Helpful Tips While Waiting for HCV Treatment (Hepatitis Foundation International) - PDF
- Hepatitis C (New Mexico AIDS Education and Training Center) Also in Spanish
- Hepatitis C and HIV (AIDS.gov)
- Hepatitis C and Incarceration (Centers for Disease Control and Prevention) - PDF Also in Spanish
- Hepatitis C: Questions to Ask Your Doctor about Treatment (Department of Veterans Affairs)
- Hepatitis C: Questions to Ask Your Doctor about Your Diagnosis (Department of Veterans Affairs)
- Hepatitis C: Sex and Sexuality (Department of Veterans Affairs)
- Travelers' Health: Hepatitis C (Centers for Disease Control and Prevention)
- Vaccinations for Adults with Hepatitis C Infection (Immunization Action Coalition) - PDF Also in Spanish

Specifics

- Hepatitis C: What Happens in End-Stage Liver Disease? (Mayo Foundation for Medical Education and Research)

Health Check Tools

- Hepatitis Risk Assessment (Centers for Disease Control and Prevention)

Statistics and Research

- Hepatitis C and Dietary Supplements: What the Science Says (National Center for Complementary and Integrative Health)
- HIV Infection Accelerates Hepatitis C-Related Liver Fibrosis (National Institute on Drug Abuse)
- Surveillance for Viral Hepatitis - United States, 2012 (Centers for Disease Control and Prevention)
- The Path to a Cure for Hepatitis C in People With HIV (National Institute of Allergy and Infectious Diseases)

Clinical Trials

- ClinicalTrials.gov: Hepatitis C (National Institutes of Health)
- Hepatitis C: Clinical Trials (Department of Veterans Affairs)

Journal Articles

- Article: Viral hepatitis: the clinical nurse specialist role.
- Article: Indian hepatitis C drug patent decision shakes public health community.

- Article: Increased T and B Regulatory Cell Function Contributes to the...
- Hepatitis C -- see more articles

Find an Expert
- Centers for Disease Control and Prevention Also in Spanish
- Hepatitis Foundation International
- National Institute of Allergy and Infectious Diseases
- National Institute of Diabetes and Digestive and Kidney Diseases

Children
- Hepatitis (Nemours Foundation) Also in Spanish
- What is Hepatitis C and Why Should I Be Concerned about It? (American Academy of Pediatrics) Also in Spanish
- Hepatitis (Nemours Foundation) For Teenagers

Patient Handouts
- Hepatitis C -- children Also in Spanish
- Hepatitis C Also in Spanish
- Hepatitis virus panel Also in Spanish
- Preventing hepatitis B or C Also in Spanish
- What I Need to Know about Hepatitis C (National Institute of Diabetes and Digestive and Kidney Diseases) Also in Spanish

Online Chat Groups and Message Boards:
These sites are good places to share information and ideas with others interested in the Hepatitis C disease, treatment options, treatment experiences and related issues. Many of these sites have monitors who supervise the conversation and will remove anyone who does not respect proper internet

protocol and decorum. In some cases you will have to submit your contact information and be approved before you can participate.

Main Websites
Hepatitis Central
Hep C Friends
HepC Net Forum
http://www.medhelp.org/forums/Hepatitis-C/show/75

HepC Nomads Forum
http://hepcnomads.co.uk/phpBB3/index.php

Hepatitis C Kids Support Forum
http://hepatitisckids.freeforums.org/index.php

Janis and Friends Hep C Forum
http://forums.delphiforums.com/n/main.asp?webtag=friendship7&nav=start&prettyurl=%2Ffriendship7&gid=2088276570

Hep C New Drug Research Chat Room
https://hepatitiscnewdrugs.blogspot.com/2010/10/support-hep-c-chat-room.html

Daily Strength Support Group
https://www.dailystrength.org/group/hepatitis-c

Hepatitis C Community
http://www.medhelp.org/forums/Hepatitis-C/show/75

HEP Forums
https://forums.hepmag.com/index.php?topic=2950.0

Great source for the latest information about buying generic HCV drugs overseas is **Greg Jefferys Blog:** <u>http://hepatitisctreatment.homestead.com/index.html</u>

In person geographical Hep C support groups by state:
http://www.hepatitiscentral.com/hcv/support/

http://Facebook.com also has a numbes of member groups you must apply to and be accepted by a moderator. These are subject to change at any time and some of them may be monitored or supported by pharmaceutical manufacturers.

New rooms and support groups pop up all the time. To find a fresh list, search Google using key words: **Hepatitis C + chat + support.**

<u>**National / International HCV Organizations**</u>:
These organizations provide information, treatment options, co-pay assistance, or otherwise address salient issues surrounding the Hep C epidemic and its cure. Their websites provide educational materials, support contact information and links to many other local, regional, national and international organizations throughout the world.

American Association for the Study of Liver Diseases
AASLD is the leading organization of scientists and health care professionals committed to preventing and curing liver disease. We foster research that leads to improved treatment options for millions of liver disease patients. We advance the science and practice of hepatology through educational

conferences, training programs, professional publications, and partnerships with government agencies and sister societies. http://www.aasld.org/

American Liver Foundation: Created in 1976 by the American Association for the Study of Liver Disease (AASLD), takes a leadership role in advocating on behalf of the millions of Americans living with liver disease and their families by facilitate, while promoting education, support and research for the prevention, treatment and cure of liver disease. http://www.liverfoundation.org/

Bonnie Morgan Foundation: Our goal is to assist patients living with chronic Hepatitis C and patients post-transplant through Charitable donations in paying their share of prescription drug co-payments and deductibles. We want to reduce the financial stress the patients needs to deal with and then they can pay more attention on their heath. http://www.notwithoutafight.org/

Center for the Study of Hep C: New York City's Center for the Study of Hepatitis C, is the only comprehensive, multidisciplinary center dedicated to the study of HCV and hepatic disease in the tri-state area, where prominent scientists and dedicated physicians to work together to understand HCV infection, to effectively manage its associated liver disease, and to develop new treatments for HCV-infected patients. http://www.hepccenter.org/

Clinical Trials: A service of the U. S. National Institutes of Health, this website is a registry and results database of publicly and privately supported clinical studies of human participants conducted around the world. Clinical trials may compare a new medical approach to a standard one that is already available, to a placebo that contains no active ingredients, or to no intervention. https://clinicaltrials.gov/

Department of Veterans Affairs: The Department of Veterans Affairs (VA) leads the country in hepatitis screening, testing, treatment, research and prevention. This site provides information both for health care providers and for Veterans and the public.
http://www.hepatitis.va.gov/

HCV Advocate: The Hepatitis C Support Project (HCSP) is a registered non-profit organization founded in 1997 by Alan Franciscus and other HCV positive individuals to address the lack of education, support, and services available at that time for the HCV population. http://hcvadvocate.org/

Hepatitis C Association: The focus of the Hepatitis C Association is to educate the public, both patients and medical providers, about hepatitis C virus through educational programs and support materials, and, through Help-4-Hep a peer-operated toll-free support line.
http://www.hepcassoc.org/

Hepatitis Foundation International: HFI provides outreach, education, linkages to care and other assistance for people at risk for and those that suffer from hepatitis and other liver disease while offering continuing education for health care professionals, conducting research; and implementing

community outreach on a national and global scale.
http://hepatitisfoundation.org/

San Francisco Hepatitis C Task Force: Their mission includes: promoting better understanding and awareness about the impact of hepatitis C on San Francisco and its residents; developing better surveillance and reporting of hepatitis C; improving access to care and support services, and increase quality of life for people with hepatitis C; and making hepatitis C testing widely available and accessible.
http://www.sfhepc.org

World Hepatitis Alliance: The World Hepatitis Alliance is a not-for-profit international umbrella Non-Governmental Organisation (NGO). Our membership is composed of over 220 organisations who work in the field of viral hepatitis, representing every region of the world accessible. View the interactive map. http://www.worldhepatitsalliance.org/

REFERENCES

I HAVE HEPATITIS C

1. Lab Tests Online. (2016). *Liver Panel.* Retrieved 08/07/16 from: https://labtestsonline.org/understanding/analytes/liver-panel/tab/test?gclid=CKTitsa8r84 CFQGQaQodGQECXQ

2. Kahn, A. (2015). *Hepatic Encephalopathy.* Retrieved 08/25/16 from: http://www.healthline.com/health/hepatic-encephalopathy-2

WHAT IS HEPATITIS C?

1. World Health Organization. (2016). *Hepatitis C Fact Sheet.* Retrieved 08/09/16 from: http://www.who.int/mediacentre/factsheets/fs164/en/

2. Centers for Disease Control and Prevention. (2016). *Hepatitis C FAQs for the Public.* Retrieved 08/08/16 from: http://www.cdc.gov/hepatitis/hcv/cfaq.htm

3. Childers, L. (2016). *How Naomi Judd Conquered Hepatitis C, a Liver Condition.* Retrieved 08/10/16 from: http://www.lifescript.com/health/centers/hepatitis_c/articles/

4. Access Hollywood. (2006). *Steven Tyler Reveals battle with Hepatitis C.* Retrieved 08/11/16 from: http://www.today.com/id/15020874/ns/today-today_entertainment/t/steven-tyler-reveals-battle-hepatitis-c/#.V6xOieLD_L8

5. Fisher, L. (2015). *Pamela Anderson Says She's 'Cured' of Hepatitis C.* Retrieved 08/11/16 from: http://abcnews.go.com/Entertainment/pamela-anderson-shes-cured-hepatitis/story?id=35074396

6. Dobuzinskis, A. (2011). *Jim Nabors hospitalized with throat infection.* Retrieved 08/11/16 from: http://www.reuters.com/article/us-jimnabors-idUSTRE76I72F20110720

7. Wikipedia. (2016). *List of people with hepatitis C.* Retrieved 08/11/16 from: https://en.wikipedia.org/wiki/List_of_people_with_hepatitis_C#cite_note-17

8. Christiansen, R. (1987). *Comedic Actor Danny Kaye, 74.* Retrieved 08/11/16 from: http://articles.chicagotribune.com/1987-03-04/news/8701170650_1_mr-kaye-hepatitis-television

9. Severo, R. (2007). *Evel Knievel, 69, Daredevil on a Motorcycle, Dies.* Retrieved 08/11/16 from: http://www.nytimes.com/2007/12/01/us/01knievel.html?_r=3&adxnnl=1&oref=slogin%20&adxnnlx=1217021925-DxBNjIqmtilYK/VVuxLD7g&pagewanted=all

10. CNN.com. (1998). *Autopsy confirms Ray died of liver failure.* Retrieved 08/11/16 from: http://www.cnn.com/US/9804/24/ray.autopsy.pm/

11. Wilson, E. (2010). *Robert Schimmel, Comic, Dies at 60.* Retrieved 08/11/16 from: http://www.nytimes.com/2010/09/05/arts/television/05schimmel.html?_r=0

12. Mclellan, D. (2004). *Hubert Selby Jr., 75; Wrote Existential Novels.* Retrieved 08/11/16 from: http://articles.latimes.com/2004/apr/28/local/me-selby28

13. Lehmann-Haupt, C. (2001). *Ken Kesey, Author of 'Cuckoo's Nest,' Who Defined the Psychedelic Era, Dies at 66.* Retrieved 08/11/16 from: http://www.nytimes.com/2001/11/11/nyregion/ken-kesey-author-of-cuckoo-s-nest-who-defined-the-psychedelic-era-dies-at-66.html

14. Cohn, Nik (2005). *Triksta: Life and Death and New Orleans Rap.* New York: Random House. p. 3. ISBN 978-1-4000-7706-9.

15. Pratt, G. (2011). *Superstar Billy Graham Made It Big in Wrestling -- Now the Steroids That Got Him There May Be Killing Him.* Retrieved 08/11/16 from: http://www.phoenixnewtimes.com/news/superstar-billy-graham-

made-it-big-in-wrestling-now-the-steroids-that-got-him-there-may-be-killing-him-6448014

16. Blair, T. (2006). *Rolf Benirschke.* Retrieved 08/11/16 from: http://www.sandiegomagazine. com/San-Diego-Magazine/November-2006/Rolf-Benirschke-with-Tom-Blair/

17. Barnes, B. (1995). *Mickey Mantle, legend of baseball, dies at 63.* Retrieved 08/11/16 from: http://www.washingtonpost.com/wp-srv/sports/longterm/memories/1995/95pass6.htm

18. Snyder, K. (2011). *Dr. Jack Kevorkian Dies at 83; A Doctor Who Helped End Lives.* Retrieved 08/11/16 from: http://www.nytimes.com/2011/06/04/us/04kevorkian.html?pagewanted=1&_r=1

19. Oppenheimer, J. (2015). *RFK Jr.: Robert F. Kennedy Jr. and the Dark Side of the Dream.* New York: St. Martin's Press. p. 252. ISBN 978-1-250-03295-9.

20. Schudel, M. (2008). *Rocky Aoki; Flashy founder of Benihana.* Retrieved 08/11/16 from: http://www.washingtonpost.com/wp-dyn/content/article/2008/07/11/AR2008071103151.html

21. Fox News. (2011). *Music Legends Fight the Stigma of Hepatitis C With New Campaign.* Retrieved 08/11/16 from: http://www.foxnews.com/health/2011/07/28/music-legends-fight-stigma-hepatitis-c-with-new-campaign.print.html#

22. Davis, C. P. (2016). *Viral Hepatitis A, B, C, D, E.* Retrieved 08/08/16 from: http://www.medicinenet.com/viral_hepatitis/article.htm

23. Franciscus, A. (2016). *A Brief History of Hepatitis C.* Retrieved 08/15/16 from: http://hcvadvocate.org/hepatitis/factsheets_pdf/Brief_History_HCV.pdf

24. Immunization Action Coalition. (2014). *Hepatitis A, B, and C: Learn the Difference. Retrieved* 08/08/16 from: www.immune.org/catg.d/p4075.pdf

25. Smith, D. B., Bukh, J., Kuiken, C., Muerhoff, A. S., Rice, C. M., Stapleton, J. T., & Simmonds, P. (2014). Expanded Classification of Hepatitis C Virus Into 7 Genotypes and 67 Subtypes: Updated Criteria and Genotype Assignment Web Resource. *Hepatology, 59*(1), 318–327. http://doi.org/10.1002/hep.26744

26. Franciscus, A. (2016). *HCV Genotype, Quasispecies & Subtype.* Retrieved 08/08/16 from: http://hcvadvocate.org/hepatitis/factsheets_pdf/genotype.pdf

27. Hepatitis Central. (2016). *Genotypes explained.* Retrieved 08/08/16 from: http://www.hepatitiscentral.com/hcv/genotype/explained/

28. Messina, J. P., Humphreys, I., Flaxman, A., Brown, A., Cooke, G. S., Pybus, O. G., Barnes, E. (2015). Global distribution and prevalence of hepatitis C virus genotypes. *Hepatology.* 61(1), 77-87. doi: 10.1002/hep.27259. Retrieved 08/10/16 from: http://www.ncbi.nlm.nih.gov/pubmed/25069599

HARVONI AND OTHER HCV DRUGS

1. Franciscus, A. (2016). *A Brief History of Hepatitis C.* Retrieved 08/15/16 from: http://hcvadvocate.org/hepatitis/factsheets_pdf/Brief_History_HCV.pdf

2. Cutler, N. (2006). *Understanding Hepatitis C Interferon Therapy.* Retrieved 08/07/16 from: http://www.hepatitiscentral.com/news/understanding_h/

3. Genentech. (2016). *Pegasys® (peginterferon alfa-2a).* Retrieved 08/07/16 from: http://www.gene.com/media/product-information/pegasys

4. Genetech. (2016). Copegus. Retrieved 08/07/16 from: http://www.gene.com/download/pdf/copegus_prescribing.pdf

5. Cherney, K. (2015). *A Full List of Hepatitis C Medications.* Retrieved 08/10/16 from: Re: http://www.healthline.com/health/hepatitis-c/full-medication-list#6

6. Chopra, S., & Muir, A. J. (2016). *Treatment regimens for chronic hepatitis C virus genotype 1 infection in adults.* Retrieved 08/10/16 from: http://www.uptodate.com/contents/treatment-regimens-for-chronic-hepatitis-c-virus-genotype-1-infection-in-adults

7. Vertex Pharmaceuticals, Inc. (2013). *Incivek: Highlights of Prescribing Information.* Retrieved 08/10/16 from: http://pi.vrtx.com/files/uspi_telaprevir.pdf

8. FDA. (2013). *Telaprevir (marketed as Incivek) Information.* Retrieved 08/08/16 from: http://www.fda.gov/Drugs/DrugSafety/PostmarketDrugSafetyInformationforPatientsandProviders/ucm332743.htm

9. Helfand, C. (2014). *Sovaldi forces Incivek off the Hep C market as Vertex calls it quits.* Retrieved 08/10/16 from: http://www.fiercepharma.com/sales-and-marketing/sovaldi-forces-incivek-off-hep-c-market-as-vertex-calls-it-quits

10. Merck Sharp & Dohme Corp. (2013). *Victrelis.* Retrieved 08/10/16 from: https://www.merck.com/product/usa/pi.../v/victrelis/victrelis_pi.pdf

11. FDA. (2013). *FDA approves Victrelis for hepatitis C virus.* Retrieved 08/08/16 from: http://www.fda.gov/NewsEvents/Newsroom/Press Announcements/ucm255390.htm

12. Loftus, P. (2015). *Merck Will No Longer Sell its Victrelis Hepatitis C Drug in the U. S.* Retrieved 08/10/16 from: http://blogs.wsj.com/pharmalot/2015/01/21/merck-will-no-longer-sell-its-victrelis-hepatitis-c-drug-in-the-u-s/

13. Jassen. (2016). *Olysio.* Retrieved 08/10/16 from: https://www.olysio.com/hcp?&utm_source= google&utm_medium= cpc&utm_campaign=Olysio+HCP+-+2016&utm_content=Olysio+-+Brand&utm_term= olysio+package+insert&gclid=CLD3urDkvs4 CFQYsMgodqHUObQ&gclsrc=ds

14. FDA. (2013). *FDA approves new treatment for hepatitis C virus.* Retrieved 08/08/16 from: http://www.fda.gov/newsevents/newsroom/pressannouncements/ucm376449.htm/

15. AbbVie. (2016). *Viekira Pak.* Retrieved 08/10/16 from:
    https://www.viekira.com/

16. FDA. (2014). *FDA approves Viekira Pak to treat hepatitis C.* Retrieved
    08/10/16 from: http://www.fda.gov/NewsEvents/Newsroom/Press
    Announcements/ucm427530.htm

17. Gilead Sciences. (2013). *Solvadi.* Retrieved 08/10/16 from:
    www.gilead.com/~/media/Files/pdfs/.../liver.../sovaldi/sovaldi_pi.pdf

18. FDA. (2013). *FDA approves Sovaldi for chronic hepatitis C.* Retrieved
    08/08/16 from: http://www.fda.gov/newsevents/newsroom/pressannoun
    cements/ucm377888.htm

19. Gilead Sciences. (2016). *Harvoni gives you what you need* [click "Full
    Prescribing Information" link at top of page.] Retrieved 08/08/16 from:
    http://www.harvoni.com/taking-harvoni/treatment-with-harvoni?utm_
    medium=cpc&utm_source=google&utm_medium=cpc&utm_
    campaign=349970702&utm_term=%2Bharvoni%20%2Btreatments
    &utm_content=17561639942&gclid=COir2ZiKsc4CFZSIaQodAlMH1A&
    gclsrc=aw.ds

20. FDA. (2014). *FDA approves first combination pill to treat hepatitis C
    [Harvoni].* Retrieved 08/08/16 from: http://www.fda.gov/newsevents/
    newsroom/pressannouncements/ucm418365.htm

21. AbbVie. (2016). *Technivie.* Retrieved 08/09/16 from:
    http://www.rxabbvie.com/pdf/technivie_pi.pdf

22. FDA. (2015). *FDA approves Technivie for treatment of chronic hepatitis C
    genotype 4.* Retrieved 08/10/16 from: http://www.fda.gov/newsevents/
    newsroom/pressannouncements/ucm455857.htm

23. Bristol-Myers Squibb. (2016). *Daklinza.* Retrieved 08/09/16 from:
    http://packageinserts.bms.com/pi/pi_daklinza.pdf

24. FDA. (2015). *FDA approves new treatment for chronic hepatitis C
    genotype 3 infections. [Daklinza].* Retrieved 08/08/16 from:
    http://www.fda.gov/NewsEvents/Newsroom/ PressAnnouncements/
    ucm455888.htm

25. Merck. (2016). *Zepatier.* Retrieved 08/10/16 from:
    https://www.merck.com/product/usa/pi.../z/zepatier/zepatier_pi.pdf

26. FDA. (2016). *FDA approves Zepatier® for treatment of chronic hepatitis C genotypes 1 and 4.* Retrieved 08/10/16 from:
    http://www.fda.gov/NewsEvents/Newsroom/PressAnnouncements/ucm483828.htm

27. Gilead Sciences. (2016). *Epclusa.* Retrieved 08/10/16 from:
    https://www.epclusainfo.com/?utm_source=google&utm_medium=cpc&utm_campaign=624265620&utm_term=%2Bepclusa&utm_content=28839024654&gclid=CPH69OKCv84CFUddMgodZtUGwQ&gclsrc=ds

28. FDA. (2016). *FDA approves Epclusa for treatment of chronic Hepatitis C virus infection.* Retrieved 08/08/16 from: http://www.fda.gov/newsevents/newsroom/pressannouncements /ucm508915.htm

29. Lazarus et al. (2014). Roundtable discussion: how lessons learned from HIV can inform the global response to viral hepatitis. *BMC Infectious Diseases,* 14,(Suppl 6):S18. http://www.biomedcentral.com/1471-2334/14/S6/S18

30. Franciscus, A. (2016). *A Brief History of Hepatitis C.* Retrieved 08/15/16 from: http://hcvadvocate.org/hepatitis/factsheets_pdf/Brief_History_HCV.pdf

31. World Health Organization. (2016). *Hepatitis C.* Retrieved 08/16/16 from: http://www.who.int/mediacentre/factsheets/fs164/en/

32. Harding, A. (2016). *Pros and Cons of New Hepatitis C Drugs.* Retrieved 08/08/16 from: http://www.everydayhealth.com/news/pros-cons-new-hepatitis-treatments-patients/

GETTING APPROVED

1. Quest Diagnostics. (2016). *Hepatitis C Viral RNA, Qualitative TMA.* Retrieved 08/07/16 from:

http://www.questdiagnostics.com/testcenter/testguide.action?dc=TH_HCV_RNA_QualTMA

2. Ernst, A. (2016). *What Is Viral Load?* Retrieved 08/17/16 from: http://www.hepatitiscentral.com/ hepatitis-c/what-is-viral-load/

3. American Liver Foundation. (2015). *The Progression of Liver Disease.* Retrieved 08/07/16 from: http://www.liverfoundation.org/abouttheliver/info/progression/?o=35294&l=sem&qsrc=990&qo=serpSearchTopBox&ad=semD&ap=google.com&an=google_s&am=broad

4. Watson, S. (2015). *Understanding Hepatitis C from Diagnosis to Stage 4.* Retrieved 08/07/16 from: http://www.healthline.com/health/stage-4-hepatitis-c#Overview1

5. Hepatitis Central. (2016). *What is Hepatic Encephalopathy?* Retrieved 08/25/16 from: http://www.hepatitiscentral.com/hcv/whatis/encephalopathy/

6. Smith, P. (2016). *How I Got the $84,000 Hepatitis C Drug for $1500 by Buying it from India.* Retrieved 08/17/16 from: http://www.alternet.org/personal-health/84000-hep-c-drug-only-1500

7. O'Donnell, K. (2013). *Buying Prescription Drugs Online Without Getting Burned.* Retrieved 08/17/16 from: http://www.bloomberg.com/news/articles/2013-08-02/buying-prescription-drugs-online-without-getting-burned

8. Staton, T. (2015). *Hep C drug tourism has begun as patients seek Harvoni, Sovaldi overseas.* Retrieved 08/15/16 from: http://www.fiercepharma.com/sales-and-marketing/hep-c-drug-tourism-has-begun-as-patients-seek-harvoni-sovaldi-overseas

9. Pettypiece, S. & Gokhale, K. (2015). *Patients Get Extreme to Obtain Hepatitis Drug That's 1% the Cost Outside U.S.* Retrieved 08/15/16 from: http://www.bloomberg.com/news/articles/2015-06-01/hepatitis-cruise-india-trips-among-plans-to-save-on-1-000-pill

10. Harvoni.com. (2016). *Eligible patients may pay no more than $5 per co-pay for HARVONI.* Retrieved 08/15/16 from: https://www.harvoni.com/support-and-savings/co-pay-coupon-registration

11. AbbVie. (2016). *Nurse Connectors can help you connect with the right resources.* Retrieved 08/18/16 from: https://www.viekira.com/patient-support/financial-resources

12. Associated Press. (2016). *Gilead ordered to pay Merck $200M for patent infringement.* Retrieved 08/17/16 from: http://www.cnbc.com/2016/03/25/gilead-ordered-to-pay-merck-200m-for-patent-infringement.html

13. Freyer, F. (2016). *Hepatitis C drug costs leave many without care.* Retrieved 08/15/16 from: https://stepuptohepco.wordpress.com/2016/04/18/hepatitis-c-drug-costs-leave-many-without-care/

14. Freyer, F. (2016). *Hepatitis C patients often have to get sicker before insurance will pay for drugs.* Retrieved 08/15/16 from: https://www.bostonglobe.com/metro/2016/04/18/insurers-balk-paying-for-hepatitis-drugs/M9Iv0SZcMhHuw1ek3zclLL/story.html#comments

15. Salzman, S. (2015). *How insurance providers deny hepatitis C patients lifesaving drugs.* Retrieved 08/15/16 from: http://america.aljazeera.com/articles/2015/10/16/insurance-providers-deny-hepatitis-drugs.html

16. Lazarus et al. (2014). Roundtable discussion: how lessons learned from HIV can inform the global response to viral hepatitis. *BMC Infectious Diseases,* 14, (Suppl 6):S18. Retrieved 08/15/16 from: http://www.biomedcentral.com/1471-2334/14/S6/S18

17. CDC. (2016). *Polio Elimination in the United States.* Retrieved 08/17/16 from: https://www.cdc.gov/polio/us/index.html

18. Huwart, L. et al. (2008). Magnetic Resonance Elastography for the Noninvasive Staging of Liver. *Gastroenterology, 135*(1), 32–40. Retrieved 08/07/16 from: http://www.gastrojournal.org/article/ S0016-5085(08)00572-6/abstract

PRE-TREATMENT PREPARATION

1. Jeanne, H. (2004). *The Hepatitis C Cookbook.* Nashville, TN: Cumberland House. ISBN 1-58182-418-1

2. Hepatitis Central. (2016). *5 Rules of the Anti-Inflammatory Diet.* Retrieved from: http://www.hepatitiscentral.com/news/5-rules-of-the-anti-inflammatory-diet/?eml=hepcen252

THE FIRST WEEK – Fears and Worries

1. Bliss, S. (2016). *Harvoni and Alcohol: Is It Safe?* Retrieved 08/20/16 from: http://www.healthline.com/health/hepatitis-c/harvoni-alcohol#Harvonioverview1

WEEKS 2 – 4: Typical Side Effects

1. Dartmouth Medical School. (2016). *Strategies to beat the host.* Retrieved 08/20/16 from: http://www.epidemic.org/thefacts/viruses/strategiesToBeatTheHost/

2. Cutler, N. (2007). *How Hepatitis C Can Affect a Patient's Sex Life.* Retrieved 08/12/16 from: http://www.hepatitiscentral.com/news/how_hepatitis_c/

3. Cutler, N. (2011). *Hepatitis C Lifestyle Management: Get Your Sexy Back.* Retrieved 08/12/16 from: http://www.hepatitiscentral.com/news/hepatitis_c_lif/

4. Nordqvist, C. (2016). *What Are Electrolytes? What Causes Electrolyte Imbalance?* Retrieved 09/21/16 from: http://www.medicalnewstoday.com/articles/153188.php

5. Porter, L. K. (2014). *Harvoni and Headaches: Why Acetaminophen is Usually the Best Remedy.* Retrieved 08/21/16 from: https://www.hepmag.com/blog/harvoni-and-headache-1

6. Cutler, N. (2007). *Pain Relievers and Hepatitis C.* Retrieved 08/21/16 from: http://www.hepatitiscentral.com/news/is_there_pain_r/

WEEKS 5 – 12: *Good Days and Bad Days*

1. Harvoni. (2016). *Adverse reactions (all grades) reported in .5% of subjects receiving 8, 12, or 24 weeks of treatment with HARVONI.* Retrieved 08/20/16 from: http://hcp.harvoni.com/?evo_source= HARVONI-V2&evo_tracker=dXRtX21lZGl1bT1jcGMsY3Bj JnV0bV9zb3VyY2U9Z 29vZ2xlJnV0bV9jY W1w YWlnbj0Zn Dk5NzA3MDImdXRtX3Rlcm09K2hhcnZvbmkmdXRtX2NvbnRlbnQ9 MTc1NjE2Mzc3ODI=

POST TREATMENT – What Next

1. Cherney, K. (2014). *Can Hepatitis C Cause Kidney Failure?* Retrieved 08/21/16 from: http://www.healthline.com/health-slideshow/hepatitis-c-kidney-failure#5

2. Palmer, E. (2015). *Gilead warns of fatal reaction to Sovaldi, Harvoni and heart drug.* Retrieved 08/25/16 from: http://www.fiercepharma.com/regulatory/gilead-warns-of-fatal-reaction-to-sovaldi-harvoni-and-heart-drug

3. Gilead. (2015). *Important Drug Warning.* Retrieved 08/21/16 from: http://freepdfhosting.com/47b90580b3.pdf

4. FDA. (2015). *FDA Drug Safety Communication: FDA warns of serious slowing of the heart rate when antiarrhythmic drug amiodarone is used with hepatitis C treatments containing sofosbuvir (Harvoni) or Sovaldi in combination with another Direct Acting Antiviral drug.* Retrieved 08/25/16 from: http://www.fda.gov/Drugs/DrugSafety/ucm439484.htm

5. U. S. National Library of Medicine. (2016). *Amiodarone.* Retrieved 08/25/16 from: https://medlineplus.gov/druginfo/meds/a687009.html

6. Catie. (2016). *Harvoni (ledipasvir + sofosbuvir).* Retrieved 08/21/16 from: http://www.catie.ca/sites/default/files/harvoni%20EN%2 02015%2003%2027.pdf

7. Gilead Sciences. (2016). *Harvoni gives you what you need* [click "Full Prescribing Information" link at top of page.] Retrieved 08/08/16 from: http://www.harvoni.com/taking-harvoni/treatment-with-harvoni?utm_medium=cpc&utm_source=google&utm_medium=cpc&utm_campaign=349970702&utm_term=%2Bharvoni%20%2Btreatments&utm_content=17561639942&gclid=COir2ZiKsc4CFZSIaQodAlMH1A&gclsrc=aw.ds

AFTERWARD – Am I Really Cured?

1. Daniel, C. (2016). *What Is a Sustained Virologic Response? Understanding the Clinical Definition of a Hepatitis C "Cure".* Retrieved 08/23/16 from: https://www.verywell.com/what-is-a-sustained-virologic-response-or-svr-1760132

2. Cutler, N. (2014). *After Being Cured... Can Hep C Return?* Retrieved 08/1016 from: http://www.hepatitiscentral.com/news/after-being-cured-can-hep-c-return/

3. Cutler, N. (2014). *Cured of Hepatitis C: Is There Potential to Infect Others?* Retrieved 08/2016 from: http://www.hepatitiscentral.com/news/cured-of-hepatitis-c-is-there-potential-to-infect-others/

About The Authors

Valerie and Banning Lary have been together for 30 years. Valerie's Hep C began to cause problems with her health about ten years ago and got progressively worse. She investigated the interferon / ribavirin option, but the horrendous side effects reported by others, plus the only 50% cure rate, made it undesirable. Then, a new one-a-day pill treatment option appeared on the horizon: Harvoni. As her condition worsened, her doctor got her approved for a 12-week treatment. Her viral load dropped from 4,660,000 to undetected in two weeks and remained there. Her side effects were minimal as she changed her diet, drank a lot of pure water and exercised. She kept a daily journal of her experiences which forms the backbone of this book.

Banning Lary, PhD (psychology) is certified in Choice Theory / Reality Therapy, and is an award-winning writer, editor and multimedia producer specializing in educational documentaries. His work has spread useful and practical knowledge to millions of people around the world.

www.ingramcontent.com/pod-product-compliance
Lightning Source LLC
Chambersburg PA
CBHW050006070726

47592CB00018B/1069